The text in this book presents arguments both for and against drinking. It references contemporary scientific literature in order to meet the guidelines established by the National Institute on Alcohol Abuse and Alcoholism, the Bureau of Alcohol, Tobacco and Firearms and the Federal Trade Commission for objectivity. It's purpose is to stimulate public discussion about the societal benefits of responsible drinking.

Those of us who have worked for years encouraging and supporting educational approaches to alcohol abuse prevention are grateful for Gene Ford's balanced and thoughtful book.

William Coors,
Adolph Coors Brewing Company

Ford says openly, and others privately, that they see a world-wide conspiracy whose members include anti-alcohol religious groups, do-gooder public health groups and strident social engineers.

Jonathan Susskind,
The Seattle Post Intelligencer

Ford is not a Pied Piper of the beverage alcohol industry, seeking to promote a national orgy, but one who seeks to present factual evidence of the benefits and pleasures of moderation.

Harvey Finkel, M.D.,
The Wine Educator

W9-BVM-434

In response to the Carry Nations among us, author and lecturer Gene Ford has written a comprehensive new book, *The Benefits of Moderate Drinking*. Ford reviews all the relevant literature on alcohol and human health and charges that fearmongers have exaggerated the negative effects of alcohol and buried the research demonstrating alcohol's health effects.

Richard E. Sincere,
Staten Island Eagle

On balance, Gene Ford's message is a simple one. Educate people. Thoroughly study and publicly discuss the effects of alcohol consumption, positive as well as negative. Learn the lessons of history. Teach the meaning and practice of moderation.

Paul Gregutt,
The Wine Spectator

People want to and will drink, contends Ford, but after being "browbeaten" for over a century that alcohol is "evil" they've accepted their guilt. It seems then that support for Ford's crusade will have to come from the drinking public.

Matthew Fleagle,
Washington Magazine

I wrote about Ford's magazine because his seems a lone voice in our national discussion about alcohol. Being a lone voice, however, doesn't mean you don't have some valid points.

Erik Lacitis,
The Seattle Times

The French Paradox

&

Drinking for Health

By Gene Ford

Wine Appreciation Guild
San Francisco, California

Library of Congress Cataloging-in-Publication Data

The French Paradox & Drinking for Health

Gene Ford 288 p.

Bibliography: 20 p.
Index 9 p.

1. Drinking of alcoholic beverages—United States. 2. Temperance.
3. Alcoholism—United States.

92-050710

Published by The Wine Appreciation Guild
360 Swift Avenue
South San Francisco CA 94080
www.wineappreciation.com
(800) 231-9463

Copyright Gene Ford Publications, Inc. 2003

Printed in the United States of America 10 9 8 7 6 5 4 3

ISBN 0-932664-81-4

Contents

Foreword

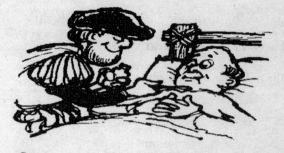

Aspirin in regular, small doses is life-giving; aspirin in episodic, large amounts is life-taking. Despite the potential for serious consequences from aspirin overdosage, the ease of maintaining the intake of a low dose has established the use of aspirin as a major advance in the prevention of heart disease.

Alcohol, like aspirin, in regular, small doses is life-giving; alcohol, like aspirin, in episodic, large doses is life-taking. Because it is very difficult to limit the intake of alcohol by the one of ten people who choose to abuse themselves or who become addicted to its effects, a broad attack upon the dangerous misuse of alcohol has been instituted.

Unfortunately, as Gene Ford has so carefully documented in this book, the well-intentioned attempt to prevent alcohol abuse threatens to restrict the healthful use of alcohol, throwing out the baby (and the parents) with the bath water.

Both the public at large and the health-care profession must continue to do everything possible to prevent alcohol abuse. At the same time, it is essential not to prohibit or impede the continued healthful consumption of moderate amounts of alcohol—the practice of the overwhelming majority of the people who drink.

There are many similarities but also some major differences between the campaign to prevent abuse but not to totally prohibit the moderate use of alcohol with the campaign to restrict but not to totally prohibit the smoking of tobacco.

The major differences between alcohol and tobacco are that tobacco has no health benefits and is many times more addictive. For good reason, all health-care professionals and the majority of the public are in favor of reasonable restrictions on tobacco use, particularly for the children who are so susceptible to becoming addicted. Few, however, want to totally prohibit the availability and use of tobacco—despite the strength of the arguments that the only way to save the 435,000 people in the nation who die each year from tobacco is to do so.

Although alcohol is much less addictive than tobacco, we must continue to protect those who are susceptible to its misuse, particularly adolescents and those who have become addicted alcohol abusers. On the other hand, we should be very careful not to frighten the majority of the population who drink moderately so that they will deny themselves and everyone else the major protection against premature heart disease from regular, moderate alcohol intake.

I am particularly upset by those health-care professionals who are unwilling to advocate healthful drinking because of their mistaken belief that any such advocacy will encourage alcohol abuse. Certainly, health-care professionals have, in general, been too timid in their campaign against tobacco. At the same time, I believe they have been too indiscriminate in their campaign against drinking. A proper balance is feasible—restricting alcohol abuse, encouraging moderate alcohol use.

This book and Gene Ford's long-time efforts should help us achieve this proper balance.

Norman M. Kaplan, M.D.

It's been written . . .

The nub of the issue: why are the healthiest, longest-lived nations on earth so panicked about their health. The central paradox of the new concern—sometimes panic—about threats to health can be stated simply.

Health is the new activism of the new class or the new religion. Second, the panic is due to the problems of presenting scientific research with all its nuances to a blip-attentive public via a sensationalist media, neither of which know or are interested in knowing much science.

Health, Lifestyle & Environment: Countering the Panic, Social Affairs Unit, London 1992

Author's statement

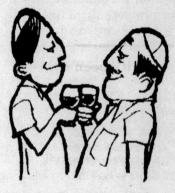

I drink to your health!

A *votre sante'. Prost. Skoal. L'Chayim.* There is hardly a language in the world in which drinking is not linked with good fortune and long life. Despite the universality of its abuse, drinking symbolizes good health and longevity in the folklore and poetry of most nations.

Last November, a *60 Minutes* airing of the "French Paradox" suggested an answer to the riddle of how the French people could eat foods thought harmful to the heart and sustain low rates of heart disease. The answer suggested was the consumption of alcohol. This book—a revision of an earlier text—reports on this *positive* science about

drinking as well as the evils of abuse. I do not
suggest that drinking is necessary or even
desirable for the maintenance of good health.
I do not promote drinking. But I do bring to
light a profound and extensive body of
research that attests that moderate drinking
itself can contribute to good heart health, to a
lessening of other diseases and that drinking
can and does contribute to general well-being.
I suggests that the real "drinking problem" is
the myth of *demon rum,* our 200 year-old
distorted way of looking at one of nature's
blessings—potable alcohol.

> *The alcohol problem, or alcohol*
> *abuse, as it is commonly under-*
> *stood and talked about today, is not*
> *a thing, or a number of things—it*
> *is a relationship. . . . This medical,*
> *scientific and popular way of view-*
> *ing alcohol is nearly 200 years old—*
> *but no more (Levine 1984).*

The control movement

The good news of drinking is little known
because of a resurgence of the 200 year-old
anti-drinking movement. I assert that the
federal goverment is leading this effort. The
movement is fostered by public health
professionals including the World Health
Organization (WHO). The goal is to reduce

per capita drinking throughout the world. This goal is based upon a research theory called the Control of Availability. It appears logical. It holds that as overall drinking goes down, the abusive minority will also drink less. Sounds good, but it doesn't work. Abusers are not logical.

However, if you accept the control theory, punitive control restrictions can be justified to make that reduction including the defamation of even moderate, responsible drinking. Neodry proponents associate wholesome food drinks with unhealthy tobacco and illicit street drugs. They use fear—*fear* of bad health, *fear* of drunken driving, *fear* of fetal harm, *fear* of despoiling youth, *fear* of cancer—to discourage any drinking.

This book ends with a vigorous challenge of our federal bureaucracy's involvement in this international neoprohibition movement. The irony (scandal) of government funding of dry programs is that beer, wine and spirits are the only commodities in our land mandated by a Constitutional Amendment. We voted *for* drinking through ratification of the Twenty-First Amendment.

Since this popular mandate has never been rescinded, it is unconstitutional for national and state governments to destroy the liquor trade. It is certainly of questionable ethics to tax alcoholic beverages outrageously and then use those very dollars to destroy the industries from which the taxes arise.

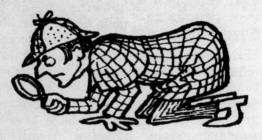

Inspecting the science

A medical researcher familiar with research jargon should have written this book. It won't happen in the present climate. Drinking is not a topic which invites open and free discussion today in grant-giving agencies, or one likely to add luster to a developing research career. The cards are stacked against positive drinking research. Correct "research thinking" is anti-drinking.

The Department of Health and Human Services (HHS), the National Institute on Alcohol Abuse and Alcoholism (NIAAA), the Alcohol Drug and Mental Health Administration (ADAMHA), the Office of Substance Abuse Prevention (OSAP) and other agencies now endorse the Control of

Availability programs. The bureaucrats don't
like drinking.

Both the Reagan and Bush
administrations have been indifferent (at
best) toward this growing anti-drinking
policy within the public health bureaus. It
was Otis Bowen, a former HHS Secretary,
that instituted the infamous "alcohol and
other drugs" theme into governmental
language and practice in 1987. The January
1988 issue of *ADAMHA NEWS* reported on a
speech by Dr. Ian MacDonald, White House
advisor on alcohol affairs. MacDonald
complained that emphasis on street drugs
"has slighted the role of alcohol as the number
one drug of abuse." He urged federal and state
administrators to *emphasize alcohol*
problems:

> *Use the term "alcohol and other*
> *drug abuse" rather than "substance*
> *abuse" in HHS publications . . .*
> *NIAAA's budget has increased by*
> *33 percent and the majority of the*
> *$163 million in funds earmarked*
> *for drug abuse treatment by*
> *ADAMHA will be received by*
> *alcoholism and alcohol abuse*
> *programs.*

With substantial increases in funding, OSAP now supports groups that are openly hostile to any drinking. There is a concerted effort to shift public attention in the War on Drugs to attacks on drinking. OSAP is establishing and manipulating political action committees to promote control legislation. Many agencies like the Alcohol Policy Conference (APC), the National Conference on Alcoholism and Drug Dependence (NCADD) and the National Coalition to Prevent Impaired Driving (NCPID) benefit from OSAP grants. NCPID asks in its membership application:

> *In the past three years, has your organization (or you as an individual) received direct or in-kind contributions from the alcoholic beverage industry or a member thereof (including producers, distributors, wholesalers, or retailers of alcoholic beverages, or their corporate affiliates)?*

If you believe that McCarthyism went out of vogue in the 1950s, you haven't been exposed to the cold hand of federal neoprohibition. What business is it of NCPID whether I have a *relationship* with a licensed beverage firm. In fact I do. I receive a monthly pension check from a winery and I accept industry advertising in my publication *The Moderation Reader*. As a consequence, I have been excluded from membership in NCPID, even though it receives federal backing.

In addition to the disclaimer above, NCPID applicants must *sign a pledge* to support the ten "Summary Recommendations" of ex-Surgeon General C. Everett Koop's impaired driving workshop. These include restraints on fair trade such as punitive taxation and elimination of product advertising. All neodry political goals.. It is illegal to use federal funds to underwrite political action campaigns.

Restrictions on the NCPID membership application disqualify thousands of experienced and willing industry volunteers who have worked for decades to assure safe roadways. We should not be asked whether we drink or whether we associate with others who drink, but whether we support workable programs for the prevention of impaired driving. That should be the goal of NCPID but its hidden agenda is the neodry agenda.

The National Beer Wholesalers Association recently enlisted over 100 members of Congress to seek a study of OSAP's political activities by the Government Accounting Office (GAO). The study will discern whether OSAP is using federal funds

to further legislation. Not surprisingly,
NCPID, Mothers Against Drunk Driving, the
Advocacy Institute and others in the
anti-drinking lobby have initiated a
campaign to derail the GAO study.
Representatives who signed the request are
urged to recant. One insulting letter asks the
members to drop their support because their
name undoubtedly "appeared on this letter
because of an administrative error . . ."

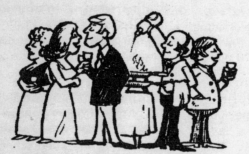

The universal tranquilizer

Of course moderate drinking is *good for a
person* in the same manner that aspirin or
beef—in moderate amounts—add to the
well-being of an individual. Ethyl alcohol
provides calories and relieves stress. These
physiological factors alone justify its
moderate usage. Of course immoderate
drinking contributes massively to personal,
family and societal problems.

Ethyl alcohol (a product of natural fermentation) is indeed a psychoactive drug—as claimed by neo-prohibitionists. But the drys never report on the very specific and positive pharmacological effects of ethyl alcohol. In moderate drinking, wine, beer and distilled spirits are efficient sources of non-carbohydrate energy. Drinking helps us celebrate births, mourn the dead and extol human achievements. Drinks containing alcohol are used to christen ships and to solemnize international treaties. In the words of philosopher William James, drinking "stimulates the mystical facilities of human nature which are crushed to earth by the cold facts of the sober hour."

Though a tranquilizer, alcohol temporarily *stimulates* human activity through the release of inhibitions. Moderate drinking enhances the human appetite by stimulating the secretion of gastric juices, particularly among the aging. Research has shown that alcohol aids in catalyzing additional vitamins and minerals from the diet. Ethanol's tranquilizing properties reduce human tensions.

Most forms of licensed beverages also contain trace amounts of minerals and vitamins which add to the well-being of the user. Alcohol is the one, holy, catholic and universal social lubricant.

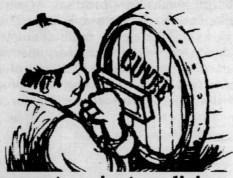

The most ancient medicine

Beverages containing alcohol are among the oldest of human medicines. Over half of the hospitals in America today make drinks available to their patients. Surveys indicate that stays in hospital for similar illnesses are shorter among drinking patients.

The Roman physician Galen called wine the nurse of old age. Its anesthetic properties temper human aches and pains in the same manner as aspirin. Because it dilates capillaries, ethanol helps bring oxygen to the body's extremities. Studies across the globe observe that moderate drinkers have fewer heart attacks and other common illnesses. Statistically, moderate drinkers live longer and experience fewer hospitalizations.

In the forms in which we ingest them, licensed beverages are simple foods. They add to our well-being as caloric energy, as ancillary sources of vitamins and minerals and as therapeutic drugs. The long standing theme used by Coca Cola is quite appropriate to drinking—*the pause that refreshes.*

Coca Cola refreshes using carbonated water and two popular drugs—caffeine and sugar. Wine is fruit juice and beer is liquid cereal. Each has a small portion of another popular drug—ethyl alcohol. Distilled spirits are often served in carbonated beverages or in fruit juices which refresh the body while adding trace amounts of vitamins and minerals.

Aside from these bare-bones facts, there is joy, camaraderie, trust, celebration and emotional richness in the human experience because of alcohol. Drinking is not a tolerable evil. *Drinking belongs* in the human enterprise.

Drinking myths

We drink because these beverages make us feel good. Here is a favorite passage from *Fermented Food Beverages in Nutrition* (Morse 1979) that puts it all together:

> *Clearly alcohol can serve many
> purposes through its pharmaco-
> logical and symbolic charac-
> teristics. It gives pleasure, reduces
> pain, eliminates fears, raises self-
> esteem, solves conflict and so on.
> But basically the pleasurable
> experience from alcohol underlies
> all alcohol problems and perhaps
> all alcohol use. The alcoholic
> drinks to relieve tension, to
> celebrate, to become brave, to be
> sociable, to handle boredom, to
> unwind, to get drunk, to feel good,
> to drown his sorrows, to get high—
> in other words, for the same
> reasons everyone else drinks. In its
> nature and quality, however, his
> drinking has changed from that
> of a nonalcoholic.*

Every society must determine its symbolic and practical roles for drinking. Philosopher Joseph Campbell correctly notes that humans are more influenced by symbols and myths than by the real world. Unfortunately, there are few substances with more powerfully *negative* myths than drinking.

Pollster Louis Harris demonstrated the power of these negative myths. *Inside America* (Harris 1987) reports "that 32% of the nation's households have someone at home with a drinking problem" and "A high of 40% of yuppies report they have a real drinking problem." I have been unable to find any evidence in the professional literature that such high abuse numbers prevail in our nation, particularly among the yuppie generation.

Americans are beginning to *believe* the propaganda that daily drinking is tantamount to harmful drinking. A 1987 study by the Centers for Disease Control is typical of a calculated governmental deceit. It states the opinion of a CDC nutrition researcher (Williamson 1987):

> *It's not clear which is more harm-*
> *ful, 60 drinks in a month on three*
> *days. . . or consuming every day.*

I called Williamson to ask what proof he had that consuming every day was harmful. He cited a statement in NIAAA's *Sixth Special Report to Congress on Alcohol and Health* that two drinks a day is heavy drinking. In this manner, government propaganda feeds upon itself.

Gallup polls also reflect the consequence of the demon rum myth-making. Gallup recently reported that only 17% favor a return of prohibition, but over 75% "favor a federal law that would require TV and radio stations

carrying alcohol commercials to provide equal
time for health warning messages about
drinking." These poll responses reflect an
ambivalence. Americans want to drink but
want the media to say drinking is
unhealthful. The myths prevail. Drinking is
depicted widely as an unhealthful practice.

As a retired wine salesman, a college
teacher and and a beverage journalist, I
became concerned about this prohibitionary
drift six years ago. Since then, I have
published 34 bi-monthly journals and two
books on drinking and health and made
dozens of speeches around the country.

Among the hundreds of texts and articles
on drinking I've read during this personal
odyssey, there is one book of such power and
clarity that it is a must-read for anyone
seriously interested in the drinking problem.
That is *Alcohol: The Neutral Spirit* (Berkeley
Medallion Books, New York, 1960) by Berton
Roueche'. Though out of print, the book is well
worth a library search. The author
emphasizes our pervasive and destructive
alcohol myths:

> *The popular mythology of alcohol is
> a vast and vehement book. It is also
> a book of massive durability.
> Almost every vision of alcohol that
> the human imagination has*

> *summoned up during some six*
> *thousand years of fascinated*
> *scrutiny may still be found among*
> *its pages. As a compendium of*
> *ageless error, of phantom fears and*
> *ghostlier reassurances, it probably*
> *has no equal. It is, perhaps, the*
> *classic text in the illiterature of*
> *medicine.*

Yes, the myth of demon rum is "illiterature" that is serving our nation poorly. Anti-drinking *myths* do not change the favorable *science* but they create an atmosphere of doubt about drinking.

There is no question that alcohol abuse is both universal and persistent. Hundreds of millions of dollars are invested annually around the world in research, prevention and treatment of this phenomenon. There is a profusion of science on alcohol abuse. There are tons of learned journals in my research depot—the University of Washington medical library—briming with seldom-read reports on abuse studies.

Yet there is very little meaningful research about moderate drinking. The government does not fund studies on why people consume moderately or what positive effects may flow from the practice. The entire science of drinking is blind-sided, single-focused, and abuse oriented.

Despite what the dry lobby likes to say, there are no abuse supporters. Even alcoholics regret their addictions. Beverage producers are not evil forces who promote addiction for profit. Abuse stems from a complex of human impulses. Abuse stems not from availability but from human perversity.

The benefits

As I worked my way through this cornucopia of clinical and epidemiological data on drinking, I knew I would find many evidences of drinking and good health. Even so, I was unprepared to discover the scope and universality of the *good news*. Here are random examples.

At a Washington, D.C. seminar sponsored by the Wine Institute, University of California medical professor Dr. David Whitten reported (Whitten 1987):

> *The studies that have been done show pretty clearly that the chances of suffering a cardiac death are dramatically reduced by drinking one or two glasses of wine a day or equivalent amounts of alcohol. . . .*

> *We don't have any drugs that are*
> *as good as alcohol.*

That's a good place for moderates to start. *We don't have any other drugs as good as alcohol.* Then I found a news release from the American Heart Association in 1987 about a study conducted by Dr. Charles Hennekens and associates at Harvard University. The study found something startling about drinking and the risk of coronary heart disease (Hennekens 1987):

> *Analyses showed that compared*
> *with non-drinkers, people who*
> *drank "moderate" amounts of*
> *alcohol every day—defined as two*
> *beers or wines or one mixed drink—*
> *had a 49 percent lower risk of a*
> *heart attack.*

The irony of is that Hennekens was also on the team that discovered the widely publicized benefits—a 47 percent reduction in heart attack risk—among those who ingest an aspirin every other day. The American Heart Association (AHA) funded both studies. AHA widely touted the aspirin findings and virtually ignored the alcohol results.

I called AHA and asked about its reticence to publicize with the same enthusiasm this extremely good news for the country's 130 million moderate drinkers. In a typical response, I was informed that it would be unwise to make much of the alcohol findings because of the danger of over-drinking.

The science says that abusive drinking has remained relatively constant through the last century and is predicted by NIAAA (*Epidemiological Bulletin #15* 1987) to remain relatively constant again through the 1990s. There is no significant danger that moderates will suddenly become abusers. Alcohol abuse is *endemic*, not epidemic, public health propaganda notwithstanding.

Heart data

The French paradox is a good starting point—not a destination—for a discussion of heart research. Indeed, the French paradox research is essentially a set of questions about *why* the benefits exists for the French. That they exist is not at question. Here are other convincing examples in the literature from around the world that demonstrate drinkers have less heart disease:

> ... *and alcohol intake (inversely) remained as a significant predictor of coronary heart disease. (Yano, Honolulu, 1988).*

*The principal finding is a strong
and specific negative association
between ischaemic heart disease
deaths and alcohol consumption
wholly attributable to wine
consumption. (St. Leger, the
European continent, 1979).*

*Coronary heart disease. . . was
negatively associated with drinking
during the follow up. (Gordon,
Albany, New York, 1987).*

*Based on this information, it was
found that the incidence of
cardiovascular in general and
CHD (coronary heart disease) in
particular were inverseley related
to the amount of alcohol regularly
consumed. (Gordon, Framingham,
Massachusetts, 1983).*

*The consistency, strength,
specificity, dose-response, and inde-
pendence of the association between
moderate alcohol consumption and
CAD (coronary artery disease)
implies a causal relationship.
(Moore, a survey of the professional
literature since 1900, 1986).*

If Americans were made aware of these many benefits among moderate drinkers, it is obvious that many more individuals would drink moderately. Public health professionals seldom mention that the United States has fewer drinkers than nearly all industrialized nations. That's what is so threatening about the French paradox to the dry lobbies. If the research identifies moderate drinking as positive to heart health, the whole "alcohol and other drugs" house of cards comes tumbling down. It is not just another drug!

The impressive good news

Despite this government policy of de-emphasizing the positive attributes of moderate drinking, scientists keep piling up the good news. Wine, beer and spirits producers don't lack proof of benefits in the scientific literature. They lack a system to bring the data to the public. In fact, the producers are threatened by government sanctions and private law suits if they do so!

A cursory review of literature is impressive. When Longnecker and MacMahon reported in the *American Journal of Public Health* (Longnecker 1988) that a nationwide survey demonstrated that daily moderate drinkers have significantly less acute hospitalization, I was impressed. Then I came across the Wiley and Camacho (Wiley

1980), a nine year study on predictors of *good health* among 3,892 adults in Alameda, California. I was elated to find drinking high on their positive health factor list:

> *Moderate alcohol consumption*
> *(17-45 drinks per month) . . . is*
> *associated with the most favorable*
> *adjusted health scores.*

I was intrigued by another nationwide health survey, this one from Canada. Richman and Warren (Richman 1985) state:

> *Beer drinkers, in particular, varied*
> *from other consumers. They had*
> *significantly lower rates of mor-*
> *bidity than expected . . . In fact,*
> *persons who drank once a day had*
> *15 percent less disability than the*
> *general population. The data*
> *support the need to assess not only*
> *the risks of high alcohol intake, but*
> *the potential benefit of moderate*
> *alcohol intake in the general*
> *population.*

Morbidity is sickness. In these studies, daily drinkers had "significantly" less sickness. While this correlation is not proof of causality, it is impressive evidence that daily moderate drinking is not a health problem in itself.

These various studies often appear briefly in the popular media but they seldom are incorporated in the HHS publications which become the primary sources for health data. Congress did not charge the NIAAA and the other health agencies to report exclusively the *bad* news. But that's what they do.

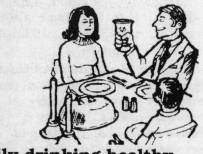

Daily drinking healthy

Most of these studies carefully distinguish between causality and correlation. It is easy to find correlations between drinking and good health. But one seldom finds drinking listed as a *causal agent* of good health in a purely scientific sense. But the correlations between responsible drinking and well-being exist strongly and they persist throughout the peer-reviewed literature of many nations.

This is remarkably true with heart disease. At the very minimum, daily drinking has no apparent physiological harm to millions of our fellow citizens. There are psychological factors in drinking that are difficult to quantify in a medical sense. These include the reduction of stress and the nurturing of human sociability. Moderate drinkers *feel* better. Government health agencies ignore these intangible benefits completely.

HHS publications are loaded with anti-drinking propaganda and frightening estimates of the costs of alcohol abuse. These "facts" are seldom submitted for publication in peer-reviewed literature. Submission of findings or statistics to professional journals helps eliminate sloppy or prejudicial work. Government agencies conduct their studies apart from professional constraints. This practice sullies all government health data.

A recent study, "The Economic Costs of Alcohol Abuse: Current Methods and Estimates" (Heien 1989), demonstrated how HHS cost estimates have major flaws:

> *This study concludes that these estimates are inaccurate and that they continually overstate actual costs. . . As a result of these considerations, the estimates lack policy relevance. . . . Based on this*

> *study of the methodology and*
> *practice of alcohol abuse estima-*
> *tion, we conclude that the estimates*
> *currently used by the federal*
> *government are flawed empirically*
> *and conceptually.*

This was devastating criticism. HHS had been estimating up to $130 billion in alcohol abuse costs. In response, HHS hired another respected expert who reported total costs closer to $50 billion. Currently the agency is ignoring this new estimate and continuing to use the fraudulent estimates.

The illicit drug linkage

How can people believe there are benefits in drinking when the federal health bureaucracy insists "alcohol is the most abused drug" in our land? Alcohol is often and tragically abused but it is far from the most abused drug. In terms of numbers of abusers, and ultimate consequences of abuse, sugar, marijuana, cigarettes and tranquilizing drugs represent more danger than alcohol.

Again, Roueche' is right on the mark:

> *Although alcohol is generally*
> *conceded a place in mid-twentieth*
> *century medicine, the position it*

> *occupies there falls somewhat short*
> *of imposing. That it has one at all,*
> *however, is something short of a*
> *triumph. It can smother pain. It*
> *can summon sleep. And it can,*
> *above all, placate the troubled*
> *spirit and rest the racing mind. . .*
> *There are other analgesics, other*
> *soporifics, and many ataractics*
> *which are not merely as good, but*
> *in almost every respect, almost*
> *immeasurably better. Their only*
> *flaw is excellence. . . They are also,*
> *unlike alcohol, incapable of giving*
> *pleasure. They can only offer the*
> *chilly charity of relief.*

I never slight the very serious health and economic problems in alcohol abuse. But I do argue that HHS must be forced to curtail its open hostility to all drinking. Only then can we establish a responsible drinking ethic which will encompass the healthful habits of the moderate majority.

No one needs to drink

No one needs to drink to lead a healthy, happy, rewarding life. This should be said over and over again, but it's not the main point. At no time in two decades of teaching, reading and writing on this subject have I counseled others to drink. Most Americans do consume alcohol, always have, and, quite likely, always will. The point is that the health and well-being of the overwhelming preponderance of drinkers is being ignored in favor of reducing the endemic abuse of a minority.

All drinkers should vigorously object to the government's insulting comparisons of responsible drinking with illicit drugging. Why should the government encumber our choices by imposing punitive taxation and laws that make purchasing inconvenient and more costly for an innocent majority?

Drinking and health faddism

The worst thing that responsible drinkers could do would be to elevate drinking to a health fad. A recent heart study reported by the American Medical Association demonstrates the silliness of selecting out single dietary panaceas.

In "Eating Nuts May Reduce the Risk of Coronary Heart Disease" (Fraser 1992), the researchers inventoried food intake of Seventh Day Adventists (a group with low heart disease) and found that the consumption of whole wheat bread and eating nuts more than five times a week was associated with lower relative risks for heart attack and fatal coronary disease. Dr. William Castelli, director of the Framingham project, criticized this study for its failure to incorporate other CHD factors such as dietary fats and cholesterol.

No matter how interesting, findings like "nuts for heart health" must be approached with caution. But it is outrageous for federal authorities to discourage research on the universally recognized benefits from drinking. One scientist told me that he has found an "alcohol wall" in funding agencies that blocks research which might yield positive factors about drinking.

In this atmosphere, it should come as no surprise that the National Institutes of Health turned down the initial proposal by Dr. Curtis Ellison to study the French Paradox (see page 59). The June issue of *The Lancet* has an article by Dr. Serge Renaud, Ellison's French counterpart on the *60 Minutes* program. This study cites "sticky platelets" as negative index potentially as important as low density lipoprotein in heart health:

> *Drugs such as aspirin that inhibit*
> *platelet aggregability protect*
> *against myocardial infarction. An*
> *increase in platelet aggregation has*
> *been significantly associated with*

> *increased prevalence and incidence
> of CHD.*

Given these promising findings and the cooperation of famed scientists from several nations like Dr. Renaud, one must question the wisdom of federal authorities in denying Ellison research funding. Congress should consider the advice which appeared in the December 1991 issue of *The Economist:*

> *Governments are right to warn
> people of risks of alcohol. They go
> wrong when they address health
> risks not by maximising the
> information but by maximising
> bossiness.*

A new national perspective

I don't pretend to have all the answers, but I certainly raise some important questions about our public health bureaucracy. To maintain, as that bureaucracy does, that drinking is always "risk-taking" is poppycock. There is no support for this dire conclusion in the scientific literature. The NIAAA itself forecasts no major changes in the 1990s in rates of addiction. We have about the same percent of abusers today as in the 1860s.

I present both the good and bad news, but
it is my purpose in this book to press the
interests of moderates. I seek to end the
"alcohol and other drugs" policy which insults
moderates   and   is   lousy   science.
Neoprohibition is as bad for society as was old
prohibition. It promises a lot but it delivers
economic chaos and social disintegration.

The alternative

There is an alternative to this public health
radicalism. It lies in the responsible drinking
philosophy espoused in the 1970s *Task Force
on Responsible Decisions About Alcohol*. This
study by the Education Commission of the
States (ECS) is the only comprehensive,
broad-based study ever conducted about
drinking in our nation. It involved governors,
educators, the producing industries, and
alcoholism prevention workers. Everybody
had their say.

These findings were buried at HHS.
President Jimmy Carter adopted the ECS
report as the policy of his administration. Had
Carter been elected to a second term, it's
possible that neoprohibition would not
dominate government policy today.

Developing a public debate

The appearance of Dr. Curtis Ellison on *60 Minutes* and his speech to the Washington Press Club in May 1992 created new interest in the media about alcohol control policies. Last year, two prominent cardiologists had the temerity to speak-out about the danger of *losing the protective effects* from drinking. Dr. Arthur Klatsky, chief of cardiology at Oakland's Kaiser Permanente Hospital addressed the National Press Club. His speech "Alcohol and Cardiovascular Disorders: Abstinence May Be Hazardous to Some Persons" (Klatsky 1991). Klatsky included the following:

> *To conclude, current evidence about lighter drinking and health suggests that: (1) the case is now quite strong that, for persons at risk of coronary disease, there is an optimal amount, not just a safe amount of drinking; (2) this benefit of alcohol operates by reducing the risk of the commonest kind of heart disease—coronary heart disease; (3) we cannot yet define precisely the optimal amount of alcohol but that it is below 3 drinks a day; and (4) it doesn't seem to matter what type of alcoholic beverage is taken.*

At about the same time, Dr. Norman Kaplan (see Foreword) of the University of Texas Southwestern Medical Center was published in the *American Heart Journal* (Kaplan 1991). "Bashing booze; the danger of losing the benefits of moderate alcohol consumption" included the following statement:

> *All in all, it is not difficult to be positive about moderate consumption . . . I find nothing wrong or unhealthy about my current practice—a beer or two after a heavy tennis game or a glass or two of wine with dinner or a high ball after dinner.*

> *One last argument sometimes used against all alcohol consumption is that, even if moderate alcohol consumption is healthy, physicians cannot condone it because this condones heavier use and may even encourage those who now drink in moderation to become addicted abusers.*

> *To this I say "Baloney!"*

So do I.

The French paradox raises questions about anti-drinking policies in America's public health establishment. But remember the alternative. The ECS recommendations form a workable base for the development of a national consensus on responsible drinking.

If, after reading this book, you agree that government should represent moderates as well as abusers, join me in a grass roots movement sponsored by the *Moderation Reader* to end our two-century long winter of alcohol ambivalence. The first steps will be to lobby Congress to (1) direct HHS to drop its "alcohol and other drugs" policies; (2) to initiate research and funding for programs which explore the benefits of responsible drinking as well as the causes of abuse; (3) to adopt the ECS recommendations looking to a new national consensus on responsible drinking.

To your health. Moderately!

Gene Ford

Moderation Reader
4714 N.E 50th Street,
Seattle, Washington 98105-2908

Part I

The

French

Paradox

Chapter 1

Qu'est-ce que le paradoxe francais?

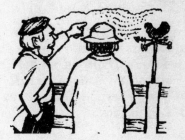

On November 17, 1991 the earth moved. On that night, 20 million Americans snuggled-in to watch the nation's favorite news/entertainment show *60 Minutes*. For the ensuing twenty minutes, Americans were shocked into a realization that there may be something good about drinking.

Here is a brief look at what host Morley Safer discovered in discussing diet and drinking in France with Boston University Medical School's epidemiologist Dr. R. Curtis Ellison and Dr. Serge Renaud. Renaud is a prominent French epidemiologist and member of INSERM, the French counterpart to our own National Institutes of Health.

Safer interviewed the doctors and other Francophile authorities and consumers.

What they discussed was a health puzzle—a paradox—in which the French smoke, lack exercise and have a diet rich in fatty foods thought bad for the heart. Yet they have remarkably low rates of heart disease.

The idea of a "French Paradox" was introduced into popular American media the year before in a serious yet delightful article in the May/June issue of *Health* (formerly *In Health*) by Edward Dolnick appropriately titled "Le Paradoxe Francaise."

> *Paris—La Coupole restaurant is jammed and, what with the noise and the difficulty of troweling just the right amount of **pate** onto my grilled bread, I'm having a hard time making out what Jacques Richard is saying. Doctor Richard, the reigning authority on heart disease rates in France, has his own problems. He can't seem to decide whether he wants yet another bite of **lardons,** the fatty bacon chunks that adorn his salad, or whether he should move on to the gooey, golden yolk of his poached egg.*

*Contrary to appearances, this is
work. I've crossed the ocean to
untangle a mystery, and if anyone
can help, it's Richard. The question
is best put as a riddle: Of the
western world's industrialized
countries, which has the lowest rate
of death from heart disease?*

Oui. C'est la France. *The United
States isn't even close. In France
each year, 143 of every 100,000
middle aged men die of heart
disease, according to the World
Health Organization. In the United
States, that figure is more than
twice as high: 315. French women
do even better, with the world's
lowest rate of death from heart
disease.*

*If you look at all industrialized
countries, only Japan beats France.
Japan's good health is no surprise,
since the Japanese diet is light on
fat and heavy on rice and fish. But
despite their bad habits the French
seem to be thriving.*

*The French have dubbed their good
fortune **le paradoxe Francaise.**
(In French, even ignorance sounds*

> *eloquent.) I'd come to France to
> solve The Case of the Unclogged
> Arteries, no matter how many three-
> star restaurants the trail might
> wind through.*

What Dolnick's article went on to presume
is that the consumption of alcoholic beverages
might be responsible—to some degree—for
the better heart health of the French. That's
a presumption that flies in the face of the
anti-drinking philosophy in American public
health—particularly federal public health
agencies—and the cautious, one might even
say niggardly, recognition of the American
heart health establishment. The French
doctor expressed no doubts to Dolnick about
the alcohol protection presumption.

> *As I sit at dinner, sipping my
> vintage Sauternes, Richard
> gestures toward the pinkish slab
> of **pate** on my plate. "That's fat," he
> warns. "Not so good for you." Then,
> with a conspiratorial grin as he
> indicates my wineglass, "You'd
> better drink your wine for
> protection."*

Compare this medical opinion of alcohol as
health protector with statements by the
Department of Health and Human Services

in the latest *Report to Congress on Alcohol and Health.*

> *The question whether moderate drinking protects against coronary heart disease, a pathological condition in the arteries that supply blood to the heart muscle, continues to generate controversy. Several epidemiologic studies have reported that moderate drinking (up to one or two drinks a day) may reduce the risk of coronary heart disease below that found in abstainers (Lange and Kinnunen 1987; Klatsky 1987; Moore and Pearson 1986). . . . On the other hand, many studies have also shown the risk of coronary artery disease and coronary artery disease mortality increases with heavy drinking (Altura 1986; Moore and Pearson 1986).*

I applaud caution in medical authority. In life and death matters, I want doctors to exercise caution and conservatism—even more so when dealing with *drinking* which has a ten thousand year history of costly misuse. But I am baffled at how public health officials dismiss a ten thousand year recorded history of alcohol as a medicine. I want doctors to look at the complete record and then make informed judgments. A characteristic which American public health officials largely ignore.

If there were even the remotest chance—and the odds are far from remote in the research—that moderate consumption could be a factor in *lowering* heart disease, public health officials should be expected to want to learn more about that possibility.

The opposite prevails. Health and Human Services issued a goal document in 1990 titled *Healthy People 2000* that is openly anti-drinking. It contains no mention of drinking's positive contributions to health. One unconscionable goal is reducing per capita drinking by nearly twenty-five percent. *Reducing* a food consumed by two-thirds of the nation which may be adding to heart health. Hard to believe? Here's goal number 4.8 from *Healthy People 2000*:

> *Reduce alcohol consumption by*
> *people aged 14 and older to an*
> *annual average of no more than*
> *2 gallons of ethanol per person.*
> *(Baseline: 2.54 gallons of ethanol*
> *in 1987).*

Let us look at the danger heart disease poses as expressed in 1992 *Heart and Stroke*

Facts published by the American Heart Association.

A Life Every 34 Seconds

What's the No. 1 killer in America?
Millions of people believe it's
cancer. They're wrong.
Cardiovascular disease holds that
deadly distinction.

FACT   In 1989, heart and blood
vessel diseases killed nearly 1
million Americans, almost as many
as cancer, accidents, pneumonia,
influenza, and all other causes of
death combined.

FACT   Almost one in two
Americans dies of cardiovascular
disease.

FACT   Of the estimated 1989
ubiquitous population of about 248
million, over 69 million—more
than one in four Americans—
suffered some form of
cardiovascular disease.

The American Heart Association pamphlet shows that alcoholism does not even show up

as a major cause of death. The critical
diseases are, in this order, cardiovascular
disease and stroke, cancer, accidents, chronic
obstructive pulmonary disease, pneumonia
and influenza, suicide and AIDS. The AHA
text makes a powerful case for paying closer
attention to heart disease.

> *Make no mistake. Cancer and*
> *other diseases are a real threat.*
> *Let's put heart disease in perspec-*
> *tive. In 1989, about 497,000*
> *Americans died of cancer. In the*
> *same year, more than 21,000*
> *Americans died of AIDS. That's*
> *tragic, but the tragedy compounds*
> *if Americans focus on these dis-*
> *eases and neglect a disease that*
> *claims nearly twice as many vic-*
> *tims.*
> *Cardiovascular diseases are killers.*

As impressive as these arguments are for
heightened concentration on heart disease
factors, I wonder why the Heart Association
ignores the voluminous research on alcohol's
role in fostering good heart health. There are
but three, brief references to drinking,
nothing about its potential protective effect.
Though well over 100 million Americans
drink with some regularity, wine, beer or

spirituous liquors didn't make the roster of protective elements.

The first alcohol entry says, "Excessive alcohol intake (more than two ounces daily) raises blood pressure in some people and should be restricted." Undeniably true. Note that "two ounces"of absolute alcohol is comparable to four standard drinks. Inexplicably, no explanation is given for the limit of two ounces other than this one line in a 48 page booklet. It appears that the AHA doesn't want to discuss drinking in any meaningful way despite the fact that two-thirds of Americans consume alcohol. Obviously, they don't want to open this "can of worms."

The second mention of alcohol concerns the "Stroke Belt" of Alabama, Arkansas, Georgia, Indiana, Kentucky, Louisiana, Mississippi, North Carolina, South Carolina, Tennessee and Virginia. In assessing the risk factors for stroke, the text identifies, "excessive alcohol intake." The Heart Association chooses to ignore the widely recognized epidemiological reality that the "Stroke Belt" is the region with the lowest per capita alcohol consumption. Why isn't this health correlation mentioned by heart association officials? Is there a conspiracy of silence about drinking and health? One must wonder. Why not say so?

It can be conjectured that the *Healthy
People 2000* goal of reducing per capita
consumption to 2 gallons could induce similar
rates of stroke around the rest of the nation.
At least some consideration should be given
those moderates who may be benefiting.

The final mention of alcohol in the
American Heart Association's 1992 report is
a gratuitous, almost throwaway, paragraph
in the "Congenital Heart Disease" section.

> *Certain conditions affecting
> multiple organs, such as Down's
> syndrome, can involve the heart
> too. A high number of congenital
> heart defects also result from
> mothers' drinking too much alcohol
> or using drugs such as cocaine
> during pregnancy.*

Again, I have no quarrel with this
statement. Nothing wrong in warning women
of the consequences of overdrinking. Contrast
the studied indifference of heart benefits from
HHS and AHA publications with a recent
report from California's Wine Institute titled
Wine and the Heart.

> *In 1985, Dr. Ronald E. LaPorte
> and colleagues analyzed all major
> coronary heart disease studies and*

*published their findings in **Recent
Developments in Alcoholism.**
Dr. LaPorte concluded that,
"Alcohol consumption is related to
total mortality in a U-shaped
manner, where moderate
consumers have a reduced total
mortality compared with total non-
consumers and heavy consumers.
Clearly, the results imply that consumption, up to one or two drinks a
day is not detrimental and may, in
fact, be beneficial for longevity."*

*One of the largest studies on alco-
hol consumption and total
mortality was conducted by Professor Arthur Klatsky and colleagues
at Kaiser Permanente Hospital
Health Plan and published in the
Annals of Internal Medicine in
1981. Results of this 10-year study
showed that drinkers of "up to two
drinks per day" lived longer and
were about 27 percent less likely to
die from all causes than either
abstainers or heavy drinkers.
Klatsky concludes this increase in
longevity for the moderate drinkers
was due to lower rates of various
diseases including coronary heart*

> *disease, cancer, and respiratory*
> *diseases.*

A recent study by Professors Paolo Boffetta and Lawrence Garfinkel for the American Cancer Society was published in the July issue of *Epidemiology*. It confirms these findings. In a 12-year long prospective study involving over 200,000 men, Boffetta and Garfinkel found that subjects who had consumed moderate amounts of alcohol were less likely to die during the research period than were men who stated they did *not* consume alcohol. This positive effect was due presumably to an approximately 20 percent reduction in death from coronary heart disease.

Dr. A.S. St. Leger, from the Medical Research Council on Epidemiology United, Cardiff, England, examined heart disease rates for 18 western countries and reported his findings in *The Lancet*.

> *The analysis showed a J-shaped*
> *curve relationship between total*
> *mortality and alcohol drinking*
> *and a U-shaped curve for coronary*
> *heart disease mortality.*

It is tempting for a wine association to overstate these findings, and perhaps tempting for moderate drinkers to believe them. But that has not been the case in America. Wineries, breweries and distilleries are hindered by government from speaking freely on health issues. Yet, the most skeptical reading of the literature assures one that, at the very minimum, daily drinking is not harmful to otherwise healthy individuals. This is not the attitude of U.S. health officials today with their "alcohol and other drugs" chants, their "Just Say No" invocations, their warning labels and signs, their threats to advertising rights, and their efforts to raise "sin taxes" to confiscatory levels to breach all manner of budgetary shortfalls.

Paraphrasing a famous comic, drinking gets no *respect.* Perhaps the public's avid response to the *60 Minutes* telecast will open more public curiosity. Why are these many scientific findings about beer, wine and spirits ignored in successive *Reports to Congress on Alcohol and Health?* We could be dealing with major medical misfeasance in this failure to inform.

When considering the French diet that, as yet, the paradox simply raises a set of questions. The relationship between drinking and heart health is not fully understood by the researchers. But it is indisputable that daily drinkers (in France and in the United States) have healthier hearts than other groups and that daily drinkers enjoy longer lives with less morbidity. U.S. health officials should be allocating millions of dollars to research this puzzle. The reality is that officials discourage research on alcohol's benefits. The following chapter is taken from a speech by Dr. Curtis Ellison. It develops his research theories about the French paradox. Will the National Institutes of Health reconsider Dr. Ellison's proposal in a favorable manner? I wonder.

Dolnick's article in *Health* ends with the author expressing envy that Dr. Richard, one of France's heart experts, gets to live in a country that so favors drinking!

> *"So, should I switch to rich cheeses and cream sauces and butter and* **pate?**

> *"No, no, no, no, no! We do not yet know what is the answer, but it is not that."Richard reflects a moment, then smiles faintly. "Perhaps it is the sky, or the light over France," he suggests, and we lift our wine glasses in melancholy tribute to the abiding distinction in our fates.*

> *He* **lives** *here.*

Chapter 2

Exploring le paradoxe

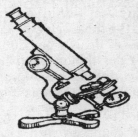

*Based on a presentation by R. Curtis Ellison,
M.D., of the Boston University School of
Medicine on May 5, 1992 to the National Press
Club, Washington, D.C.*

Epidemiological data

It is well established that the French have
much lower rates of coronary artery disease
(CAD) than Northern Europeans or
Americans. In fact, their rates are lower than
all developed nations except Japan.

In the last 10 years, CAD occurrence and
mortality rates have been monitored

according to a standardized protocol in 26 countries by a World Health Organization (WHO) project known as MONICA, for "Monitoring Trends and Determinants in Cardiovascular Disease." Data from MONICA for selected countries, and monitoring sites within certain countries, are shown in the table below of ages 35-64 years. The rates of deaths per 100,000 below are derived from tables published in 1989 in *World Health Statistics Annual* published by the World Health Organization, Geneva.

As noted in the table below, there are other European countries with rates that are not

Cardiovascular Deaths
(Per 100,000 deaths—ages 35–64)

Site	Male	Female
Japan	29	09
France	79	13
Toulouse	78	11
Spain	89	17
Italy	115	23
U.S.A.	197	61
Belfast, Ireland	348	88
Glasgow, Scotland	380	132
North Karelia	456	74

much higher than those of the French. The so-called "French Paradox" is that the French consume high levels of animal fat, similar to the intake of Northern Europe, yet have CAD rates similar to those in the Mediterranean countries, as shown in the figure above from J. L. Richard (*Les facteurs de risque coronarien. Le paradoxe francaise.* 1987; Archives Mal Coeur, Avril, 17-21).

Dietary factors

It is generally believed that the primary dietary factor related to the occurrence of CAD is saturated fat. Saturated fats in the diet come predominantly from animal products, especially meat and dairy products. Saturated fats are known to promote atherosclerosis, the underlying arterial lesion associated with CAD. When comparing populations, we see that higher saturated fat is associated with higher levels of blood cholesterol, and both are associated with higher rates of CAD. In fact, many dietary interventions designed to lower the risk of CAD are evaluated by their effects on blood cholesterol levels only, as it is difficult to judge the effects on the actual degree of atherosclerosis.

Recently, there has been a large amount of data pointing out that many dietary constituents also affect thrombosis, or blood clotting, within the arteries, a second phenomenon that contributes to CAD. It has been shown that saturated fats, polyunsaturated fats, monounsaturated fats, certain vitamins that act as anti-oxidants, and other dietary factors may play a more important role by affecting thrombosis than they do through their effects on atherosclerosis. The role of multiple dietary factors in affecting CAD risk has been discussed recently by Ulbricht and Southgate (Lancet 1991; II: 985-992).

Recent research data indicate that the French currently consume approximately 34-37% of their calories from fat, with 14-15% from saturated fat; these values are as high, or slightly higher, than recent values among Americans. We also know that, on the average, the French consume few calories from snacks (about 7.5% versus 21-25% in the U.S.). Further, while wine consumption has been decreasing among the French, especially the young people (being partially replaced by increases in the consumption of beer and spirits), the French still consume more than ten times as much wine as Americans.

My colleagues and I have been carrying out pilot work with investigators in France, Northern Ireland, and Canada, planning a project to help determine the factors that protect the French against CAD. Among the hypotheses that we plan to test are those

listed in the following table that relate to
differences in dietary practices between the
French and Americans.

> *1. The French consume more
> vegetables and fruits; foods are
> fresher; vegetables consumed raw
> or with shorter duration of cooking.*

> *2. More relaxed meals, longer
> duration of meals, less snacking
> between meals.*

> *3. Different sources of fat.*
> ✔ *Consumption of less fat from
> red meat, as meat in France is
>   much lower in fat and smaller
> portions are served;*
> ✔ *Dairy fat more in the form of
> cheese than whole milk;*
> ✔ *Use of olive oil and goose fat
> for cooking, rather than butter
>   or lard.*

> *4. Regular moderate consumption
> of alcohol with meals, especially
> wine (red wine, in particular?).*

Biologic mechanisms

Biologic mechanisms have been identified
that support some of the above hypotheses.

For example, it is well-known that fresh fruits and vegetables contain certain vitamins (vitamins C, E, beta-carotene) that serve as antioxidants. Antioxidants decrease the formation of atherosclerosis by inhibiting the uptake of LDL-cholesterol into the arterial wall. Fresher fruits and vegetables, as well as shorter duration of cooking, tend to preserve natural antioxidants. It is possible that the more gradual consumption of fats and carbohydrates may affect their absorption and metabolism, may reduce insulin levels, and/or may modify the effects of fats being absorbed on platelet function. Thus, consuming even the same amount of certain nutrients over a longer period of time could affect the action of such nutrients on the development of atherosclerosis or on thrombosis.

We know that the fatty acid content varies with different fat-containing foods. Also, some of the saturated fats (such as stearic acid) are not atherogenic. Olive oil, and to a lesser extent, goose fat, contain more monounsaturated fats than butter or other sources of saturated fat. Further, it has been postulated that the saturated fat in cheese binds differently to calcium, and may be absorbed differently, although this is yet to be confirmed in humans.

Of the hypotheses listed above, the last one (#4) has the most scientific support. There are considerable data from epidemiologic, clinical, and experimental studies which indicate that alcohol consumption lowers the risk of atherosclerosis and CAD. A number of biologic mechanisms by which alcohol affects CAD risk have been identified, as indicated below.

1. Alcohol improves blood lipid
   profile
   a. Increases HDL-cholesterol
   b. Decreases LDL-cholesterol

2. Alcohol decreases thrombosis
   a. Decreases platelet
      aggregation
   b. Decreases fibrinogen
   c. Increases fibrinolysis

3. Alcohol reduces the reaction
   to stress
   a. Reduces coronary spasm
   b. Increases coronary blood flow
   c. Reduces increase in blood
      pressure

Spirits, beer and wine

There has recently been considerable debate as to whether wine, especially red wine, protects against CAD more than other types of alcoholic beverages. Scientific data are not yet available to answer this question completely. In most cross-cultural studies, populations that normally consume wine have much lower rates of CAD than those that normally consume beer or spirits. However, consumption patterns (alcohol consumed with meals or on an empty stomach, amount consumed at one time, daily consumption versus binge-drinking, etc.) may not be the same for different beverages.

In intervention studies in humans and animals, data are accumulating that some active substances other than alcohol that are present in wine, especially in red wine, may be playing a role in the prevention of CAD. For example, Seigneur et al. (*Journal of Applied Cardiology* 1990;5:215-222) recently showed beneficial effects on platelets from red wine (but not from white wine or an ethanol solution) among healthy adult males. Data from limited studies in rabbits also support a more marked effect of wine than of other alcoholic beverages (Klurfeld & Kritchevsky, Exp & Molec Pathol, 1981;34:62-71).

Organic compounds involved

In addition to alcohol, there are hundreds of organic compounds in wine that may play a role in reducing the risk of CAD. One such compound that has recently received considerable attention is a phenolic compound known as resveratrol. Resveratrol is a naturally occurring fungicide that is present in many plants; it is contained in large amounts in the Japanese plant known as knotweed, and is used in Japan as a folk medicine.

Resveratrol also occurs on the skins of grapes and in grape juice and wine, with the level depending on the variety of grape, the degree of stress to the vine from fungus infection, the geographic area, the vineyard, and whether or not chemical pesticides have been used to decrease the risk of plant infection (the latter reduces the "stress" from fungal infection and thus the level of resveratrol). Further, resveratrol levels in wine are also related to wine-making techniques, including the time that the grape skins are left in contact with the grape juice after crushing, whether or not the wine has been filtered, etc. Siemann and Creasy have discussed resveratrol in wine in an upcoming article in the *American Journal of Enology and Viticulture*. (Vol. 43, 1992, pp. 49-52).

Conclusions

There is no question that the French have much lower rates of CAD than do individuals in most of Northern Europe, North America, and most other areas of the industrialized world. Among a number of hypotheses proposed to explain this protection against heart disease are some that relate to the preservation of anti-oxidants in the foods consumed by the French (fresher fruits and vegetables, less duration of cooking), different eating patterns (longer meals, less snacking), different sources of fat (less meat, more cheese, less milk, more olive oil and goose fat), and the regular consumption of alcohol, especially red wine.

While there is scientific evidence supporting the role of alcohol in protecting against CAD, it is not clear that differences in alcohol intake are responsible for the lower rates of heart disease in the French. Further, the relative benefit of different types of alcohol is uncertain. Additional research is needed to consider jointly the large number of lifestyle and dietary patterns that may work together to protect the French. Only then will we be able to determine if there are messages from the French that may be applicable to individuals in the United States and elsewhere.

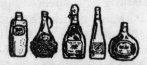

Chapter 3

Le paradoxe americain

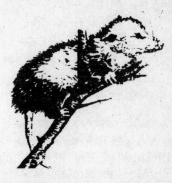

Like the humble opossum, American drinkers are figuratively up a tree.

An *American paradox* lies in the widespread ignorance of the social, economic and therapeutic benefits that result from responsible drinking. What is even more confounding is the depth of this naivete among those who grow, make and sell beer, wine and spirits. Through six years of research, writing and speechmaking around the nation about drinking and health, I remain astounded at how little liquor professionals know about the healthgiving properties in their products.

Today's "correct political thinking" today is to link drinking with drugging. This is a tortured and unrealistic linkage. Drinking is not drugging. Overdrinking's the problem.

Public health critics are already picking apart the French paradox literature as if the lower levels of heart disease in France represented a *challenge* to health rather than a hope for better health in America.

Media opening up the debate

On March 4, 1992, *New York Times* food columnist Marion Burros reported objections to the findings of the French paradox by NYU's Dr. Marion Nestle. But much more positive interest occurred in the media. The Wine Institute reports that over 200 newspaper and magazine articles featured the presumed benefits. *Vogue* and *Redbook* highlighted drinking and health in recent articles. The media suddenly seems more than interested in a new evaluation of these issues.

I warmly welcome this new curiosity in the media. Every week I get a phone call from another national columnist looking to verify one point or another about health and drinking. We may well be entering a new era in which the benefits of the existence of beer,

wine and spirits in society will be considered
along with their costs.

A balanced drinking perspective

Drinking must once again be valued in
America for what it gives as well as what it
takes. An apt comparison can be made with
the automobile. This is not a facetious
comparison. We are a nation that
passionately loves cars and brews.

Autombiles have major societal costs too.
Autos are involved in twice as many
sober-driver deaths as those related to
alcohol. Millions of Americans are
permanently maimed each year in car
mishaps in addition to those who are killed.
Cars pollute our atmosphere in a manner
that menaces survival of the species. Cars
gobble up precious natural resources. They
exact a fearsome toll in the average family
budget.

If we heeded logic alone, we would abandon
unlimited private-use of the auto in favor of
mass transportation. But, the auto *belongs* in
our culture and economy. Since we need cars
for work and play, we accept the inevitable
costs and the carnage.

Our drinks are much more intimate and
life-involving than the automobile. Yet

drinking today is perceived and discussed only in negative terms. At the birth of our nation, the *positive* aspects of drinking were a given. In Colonial days, we *loved* our drinks. Drinking *belonged* like the auto!

Just a few decades ago, when asked his opinion of bourbon by a reporter during one of his morning constitutional walks around the White House, Harry Truman responded, "Yes, please."

President Truman may have been the last politician in our nation with the courage to speak out with pride, humor and civility about his preference in social beverages. When a controversy arises about drinking today, politicians, church leaders, and titans of commerce alike distance themselves from recognition of the social, economic and health values in responsible consumption. Even executives of major firms which produce, distribute and retail wine, beer and spirits, are oddly mute.

Public health propaganda

With "booze" there are only detractors. No supporters come forth to defend a well-documented 10,000 year history of moderation. Here are three statements typical of the government propaganda drive.

Anti-drinking champion Representative Joseph Kennedy of Massachusetts portrays alcohol in speeches as the "Prince of Drugs." The congressman claims his seven year old twin children will see 100,000 beer advertisements by the age of twenty-one. From her anti-alcohol bully pulpit, Surgeon General Antonia Novello excoriates the "liquor industry" for contributing to disease, corruption of youth and death on the highways. Secretary of Health and Human Services Louis Sullivan blandly states that half of highway fatalities are "alcohol-related."

It would be virtually impossible for the Kennedy kids to view 100,000 beer ads—about 20 ads per day. Even if they did, is there anything intrinsically *evil* and *corrupting* in a beer ad? Is not beer a wholesome food product enjoyed by the majority of American adults? Kennedy doesn't complain about the thousands of automobile, aspirin or soft drink ads his kids will watch. Only "booze" ads are suspect.

Death and human misery are caused by *people* who overdrink, not by some amorphous entity which the surgeon general thinks of as the "liquor industry." The farming, manufacturing and retailing of wine, beer and spirits involves thousands of firms and millions of individual workers in dozens of trades. These Americans do not consider themselves killers or corrupters.

The number of fatalities involving intoxicated drivers is *one-third* of the total, not one-half. As a scientist, the Secretary of Health and Human Services knows the difference but continues the hyperbole.

Government's definition of *alcohol-related* itself is propagandistic itself. The National Highway Traffic Safety Administration (NHTSA) defines an alcohol-related accident as one in which the patrolman smells alcohol on the breath of any occupant of the car or the driver has a .01 BAC—the equivalence of one-third of one drink. There is enough blame to go around for drunken driving without stretching the standards beyond credulity. One-third of a drink causality is preposterous.

Where are the congressmen from California, Missouri or Kentucky to set the record straight, to question Joe Kennedy's sloppy statistics and the surgeon general's pointed harassment of industries domiciled in their states?

Beer, spirits and wine are vital commerce in more than a dozen major states. Without the farming and commercial activity and tax revenues they generate, these states would likely go bankrupt. Yet there is little response to the propaganda.

Imagine the furious public outcry from the Texas and Iowa congressional delegations if Joe Kennedy were to demean the consumption of beef. When beef was put down several years ago by similar public health pronouncements, a national Beef Council was formed and all political hell broke loose. Today, beef has regained a place of respect as a valued source of protein.

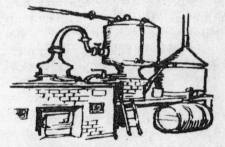

Impact of *60 Minutes*

The French paradox segment on *60 Minutes* dramatically increased sagging national wine sales. Ironically, red wines have always been a "drug" on the American wine market. Most novices prefer the softer white wines.

T*he Wine Investor* reported in June 1992
that "California is logging bigger monthly
gains than in many moons, presumably part
of the post-*60 Minutes* phenomenon . . .
shipments of French table wines are up by
9.1%. And Chile continues to roar along with
a 35.6% gain . . . our sources report
tremendous demand for Lambrusco, which
for the past few years has been in virtual
free-fall." In California, the red wine barrel
has been virtually depleted.

The response to the telecast has been
phenomenal. Hundreds of thousands of
non-wine drinkers have literally besieged
liquor outlets over the last seven months in
search of "red wines" because Morley Safer
and Dr. Curt Ellison discussed their
protective role against cardiovascular
disease. Why was the *60 Minute* coverage
such a shocker?

Public health hostility

First, there exists a pervasive
anti-drinking atmosphere within our public
health agencies. There is no other
explanation why the Department of Health
and Human Services, the American Heart
Association, the American Medical
Association and many other public and

private health organizations discourage even moderate drinking.

There are many other reasons for this institutionalized hostility to drinking. Foremost among these is the legacy of Dr. Ernest Noble, second director of National Institute on Alcohol Abuse and Alcoholism. NIAAA. Noble loaded the agency with individuals who shared his conservatism.

A second contributing factor is the very language we use to discuss the drinking. Routinely newspapers use "booze" or other disparaging words. Worse yet, the official language of research and government talks about "alcohol," not beer, wine, spirits or licensed beverages. We don't drink alcohol any more than we drink caffeine. We drink specific beverages.

Other less apparent reasons for public ambiguity lie deep in our conservative religious heritage. Rural politics also played a major role in the 1919 Prohibition. At the end of the last century, white, Protestant native American farmers and small town burghers rightfully feared the loss of political control to immigrants in the industrialized cities. Prohibition was a political act.

Today's neoprohibition movement springs from a particularly unseemly source—the public health profession. On an international level, public health operatives openly push programs which disparage responsible drinking with the mistaken hope that such efforts will solve the problems of abuse, particularly in the Third World.

Here are more reasons why neoprohibition is working in our nation.

1. The pejorative mindset

Americans still think of drink as booze. Harry Levine (*Alcohol: The Development of Sociological Perspectives on Use and Abuse,* Roman, 1991) writes "Despite the failure of constitutional prohibition, temperance culture and ideology never really lost its hold on America. Within American society alcohol remained a powerful symbol of evil, of the loss of self-control and individual responsibility."

As a moderate drinker for over half a century, I am deeply disturbed over this cultural mindset. I don't drink the "alcohol" that congressman Joseph Kennedy deplores as the "Prince of Drugs." On any day I may choose to consume a lager beer or a micro-brewed ale, a California cabernet sauvignon or a Washington chardonnay, or, quite as often, a cocktail made with a fine gin and bitters or a single malt scotch. To my mindset, each of these are legal, moral, and perfectly harmonious food beverages that add demonstrably to my chosen lifestyle.

My choices in drinks are not the desperate, haunted choices of the alcoholic who seeks and consumes "alcohol"—oblivious as to its source—to feed a compelling addiction. It is an abomination that the drinking habits of over ninety percent of Americans should be compared by government policy with the degradation and desperation of sick people—the "alcohol and other drugs" calumny.

Calling drinks booze and referring to beer, cocktails and wine as "alcohols" is not simple semantics. It is insulting and grievously damaging to the image of drinking.

2. The liability problem

American tort law is a mess. Archly-liberal legal precedents and obscenely gross damage awards in recent decades have turned our courts into Roman circuses. No one feels personal responsibility for anything anymore. Someone else—preferably a corporation with deep pockets—must bear responsibility and the financial burden for the bad luck or bad behavior of private citizens.

The waning of the ethic of personal responsibility has created liability problems for all services and sales—from physicians and restaurateurs to manufacturers of helmets and ladders. It has placed a particularly onerous burden on the licensed beverage producer. The fear of capricious lawsuits has cowed them into abject silence.

A couple of years ago, a Seattle woman bore a fetally dysfunctional child. Though she had been warned by her physician to stop drinking, she ignored the advice and ultimately brought suit against the Jim Beam Company and others demanding millions in compensation for her own behavior. Though the court held against this claim, Beam executives and managers from the other firms endured many months of personal anguish, considerable legal expenses, and a largely hostile media. It is easy to understand why industry executives choose to keep mum about alcohol and health.

3. The new social engineers

Fundamentalist churches, the Anti-Saloon League and Womens' Christian Temperance Union have stepped aside for what one professor has tabbed as new social entrepreneurs.

In the essay "The Good Life and the New Class," (*Health, Lifestyle and Environment: Countering the Panic,*1991) Irving Kristol defines a new class of social engineers who "cultivate power." Not through the normal political progression, but through clever manipulation of the media and the socio/political system.

> *They aren't interested in going into
> business, or even in making money.
> What they are interested in is
> imposing themselves on the world.
> They want power. . . They don't
> want to run things, but people.
> They want to run the people who
> run the corporations. Today they
> are doing rather well.*

The guru of engineers is Ralph Nader. One of Nader's neophytes, Michael Jacobson, runs the Center for Science in the Public Interest (CSPI). One of Jacobson's neophytes, George Hacker, runs the Advocacy Institute. In *In Pursuit of Agri-Power,* Sister Thomas More Bertels (Bertels 1988) writes, "Nader made a business of advocacy in the public interest. He formed a conglomerate of some 25 watchdog agencies each focused on a specific target." Bertels calls them "Coercive Utopians" and the "Fifth Branch of Government."

> *The public interest groups network
> with one another to an amazing de-*

gree. Even though their objectives
may be far apart, they demonstrate
a marvelous tolerance of each other.

In the pervasive negative climate, it's a
snap for Jacobson and the CSPI to pull
together impressively large coalitions such as
the over one hundred agencies which
supported warning labels on bottles.

4. Many entreprenuers at work

Armand Mauss (*Alcohol: The Development
of Sociological Perspectives on Use and Abuse,*
Roman, 1991) shows how the emerging
Naderites interlink with both public and
private anti-drinking advocacies. His article
describes each player as an "entrepreneur"
with a developed agenda but finds the new
alliance of "government" and "salvation"
entrepreneurs a powerful new social force.
"Much of the contention has focused on the
question of just what 'the problem' is. The
various interest groups attempting to define
the problem for the nation can be considered
'entrepreneurs' of different kinds."

Market Entrepreneurs

*These are the **suppliers** of the*
substances, whether in business
legally (as is the case usually for
alcohol, tobacco, and caffeine) or

*illegally (as is the case of opiates,
cocaine and the like).*

*For these entrepreneurs, the
"alcohol problem" is simply that
certain individuals drink irrespon-
sibly or for the wrong reasons . . .*

Moral Entrepreneurs

*Then there are the "moral
entrepreneurs" (as Becker called
them), who promote a variety of
normative positions on the
substance in question. . . . For
all such moral entrepreneurs, the
"alcohol problem" is found in our
rules (and/or laws) governing
the use of the substance.*

Salvation Entrepreneurs

*The success of the first two
categories—market and moral—
and, indeed, the struggle between
the two, have ironically generated
growth industries for other kinds of
entrepreneurship. One of these
might be called the "salvation
entrepreneurs" (Ralph Nader,
Michael Jacobson and George
Hacker: editor) because of the*

*close analogy they exhibit to
religious sects.*

*One sector of the salvation market
is the **prevention** sector which
includes those involved in either
public or private organizations that
are marketing prevention packages.*

*A second sector of the "salvation"
market is the **treatment** sector,
consisting of the variety of public
and private treatment and
rehabilitation programs intended
to retrieve those who have fallen
into dependency . . .*

Government Entrepreneurs

*The final general category of
entrepreneurs is "government
entrepreneurs," a market sector
consisting of all those who have
careers devoted wholly or partly to
applying government policy at the
federal, state or local levels relating
to substance use or abuse. . . For
these entrepreneurs, the "alcohol
problem" is whatever current
legislation and public policy **say** it
is, which may vary from one decade
to the next. . . However, it is important to remember also that govern-*

> *ment agencies and their personnel*
> *always have agendas of their own*
> *and thus must be regarded as*
> *entrepreneurs in their own right,*
> *as well as allies.*

The working relationships in Washington, D.C., between the private advocacies such as the Center for Science in the Public Interest, the National Council on Alcoholism and other alcohol-baiting advocacies and the government bureaucracies during the Reagan administration forged an overpowering thrust for the neo-prohibition agenda.

The "Just Say No" philosophy emerged to dominate federal policy-making. Negative presumptions became the determining factors in the distribution of federal research and project funding. State health departments, dependent largely on federal funding, began to reflect that anti-drinking bent.

Programs developed by the Office of Substance Abuse Prevention, the project arm of the drug war, and other federal agencies such as the National Commission on Drug Free Schools, and the White House Office of Drug Control Policy adopted anti-drinking programs, as did many of the old-line agencies such as the Food and Drug Administration,

National Institute on Alcohol Abuse and
Alcoholism, the Centers for Disease Control,
and even the gentle giant of alcohol control,
the Bureau of Alcohol, Tobacco and Firearms.

Indifference to health radicalism in
Congress and successive administrations fed
the ambitions of the neodrys who were then
firmly in control within government.

GAO criticizes no-use policy

The anti-drinking philosophy thrives in all
federal agencies today. A recent report to
Congress by the Government Accounting
Office (*Drug Abuse Prevention: Federal
Efforts to Identify Exemplary Programs Need
Stronger Design*, General Accounting Office,
1991) reported:

> *In developing application require-*
> *ments, OSAP and NASADAD*
> *(National Association of State*
> *Alcohol and Drug Abuse Directors)*
> *asked applicants to adhere to the*
> *no-use approach for illegal use of*
> *alcohol and other drugs.*
>
> *This requirement, like the one in*
> *the Drug-Free School Recognition*
> *Program, discourages evaluation*

and recognition of programs with
any component of responsible use
for youths, such as the 'contract for
life' used by SADD (Students
Against Driving Drunk).

GAO questions the use of a "non-federal steering committee whose purposes were not clear. This group lacked any additional information, yet their recommendations overturned 10 of the earlier reviewer's results." Not only do these agencies fund exclusively those projects which suit the neodry agenda, but they interweave known dry proponents from private advocacies on decision-making boards which award funds.

Further, they state phony conferences and symposia bringing in a stable of favored Ph.D.s and researchers who rely upon agency funding for their own projects. These government meetings specifically exclude participation by the media and the producing industries which have primary interest in abuse prevention. The industry is enemy.

Former Surgeon General C. Everett Koop staged his Workshop on Drunk Driving excluding everyone but a picked crowd which gave him his agenda. Koop then helped form the National Coalition to Prevent Impaired Driving. NCPID continues the exclusion of anyone except neodry activists.

In this negative atmosphere, the turndown of the grant application to study the French paradox by the National Institutes of Health probably came as no surprise to Dr. Curtis Ellison. Washington does not want to know anything *good* about drinking.

Consolidation of the drys

The ultimate power grab by neodry forces was announced recently by Secretary Louis Sullivan with the support of the dry bloc in Congress. It is a proposed reorganization of the vast health bureaucracy which would eliminate the Alcohol, Drug Abuse and Mental Health Administration (ADAMHA) and replace it with a Substance Abuse and Mental Health Services Administration (SAMHSA).

The reorganization itself is not nearly as important as the executive chosen to head the new department. Dr. Elaine Johnson, the former director of OSAP, has been named acting-director of ADAMHA and is heir-apparent for the reorganized agency.

Johnson has been the architect of the anti-drinking, no-use programs at OSAP. She would gain supervision of the National Institutes of Health as well as the National Institute on Alcohol Abuse and Alcoholism

consolidating the neodry philosophy through
the entire health bureaucracy.

The "salvation," "governmental" and
"prevention" entrepreneurs (in public health
sheep's clothing) will have taken charge of the
chicken coop.

Government agencies are already
exercising bully-tactics reminiscent of
Eastern European dictatorships. Recently,
the ATF threatened several tiny wineries
with the loss of their licenses if they continued
to publish material such as reprints of the *60
Minutes* telecast.

The threat is based on an ATF
interpretation that winery consumer
newsletters are "advertising" (BATF, Letter
to Leeward Winery 1992). The ATF letter
imposed blatant censorship:

> *With respect to future advertising
> (newsletters), please be advised
> that ATF provides a voluntary
> pre-clearance service for industry
> members.*

So, we see the ultimate irony of the
paradoxe Americain. The use of grossly
punitive controls and taxation on wine, beer
and spirits (sin taxes) to fund their own
demise. Private anti-drinking groups have

formed intimate working relationships with federal bureaucrats in pursuit of political programs. Neoprohibition by government fiat.

It is vital to that dry agenda that the public know as little as possible about any health attributes of drinking. The public cannot be trusted. That ls why there is so much action at ATF and HHS about wineries informing their customers about the French paradox.

ATF claims that the video program only presented one side. This implies that citizens in a free nation cannot be trusted to value research data. Cannot discern their best interests without government intervention. We used to call this thought control. It isn't any more seemly under ATF than it was under old Joe Stalin.

It's certainly paradoxical that a small group of health radicals, without a vote in any legislature, can manipulate vast and richly funded bureaus to their own political purposes.

It's a puzzlement.

Part II

Alcohol

and

Society

Chapter 4

Introduction
to drinking

Alcohol is one of the most common beverages in nature. Ethyl alcohol occurs naturally with or without the guiding hand of man as part of the ecological breakdown of plant life.

Fresh, sugar-engorged grapes ferment into wine while still hanging on their vines by the action of airborne yeast cells. As their skins burst, from the peck of a bird or the heat of the day, yeast cells gravitate from the waxy skins into the watery pulp inside. Yeast cells secrete enzymes which chemically divide each molecule of glucose or fructose sugar into equal parts of ethyl alcohol and carbon dioxide.

Alcohol the civilizing agent

The euphoria created by consuming this naturally fermented fruit made alcohol one of man's earliest culinary targets. Anthropologists hypothesize that the pursuit of a consistent supply of alcohol led to the civilization of man (Katz 1988). Wine is but one of many fermented products in nature. Other common ferments grow as molds on the skins of rotting fuits and breads. So the alcohols we consume with such gusto are formed by the ecological recycling of fruit and grain.

Beer and honey-wine (mead) were also early sources of alcohol. The sugar in a honeycomb, fallen from a tree and filled with rainwater, will ferment by the same airborne yeasts. Beer fermentation must be preceded by germination of the grain which transforms the starch to a fermentable starch called maltose.

Gifts of nature

Therefore, wine and beer were as much gifts of nature as the fruit and grains from which they were taken. Ancient man consumed thousands of edible plants, roots and seeds compared to the several hundred in use today. Long before the development of a formal cuisine, hunter-gatherers enjoyed these uniquely pleasurable and health-enhancing fermented beverages.

Anthropologists theorize that nomadic tribes gravitated to crop farming and eventually organized civil communities in order to assure a constant supply of these beverages (Kendell 1987). The wild wines or beers available were too limited and quickly depleted. This theory places alcohol among the most important and elemental forces in human society. Humans have produced alcohol as a crafted beverage for at least 8,000 years and enjoyed it in nature for many centuries more. One of the oldest written records of any civilization is a chard of pottery, depicting the brewing process.

Professor Donald Horton comments in "Alcohol Use in Primitive Societies" (Pittman and White 1992)

> *. . . alcohol appears to have the*
> *very important function throughout*
> *the world, in all kinds and all*
> *levels of human social*
> *activity, of reducing the inevitable*
> *anxieties in life. We find, in fact,*
> *that there is a general tendency for*
> *the amount of drinking, as*

> *measured by the degree of
> drunkenness obtained, to be
> roughly proportional to the
> strength of the dangers
> threatening society.*

Horton states the obvious. We drink (or
drug) too heavily when in trouble, but we also
drink moderately to reduce daily stress.
Overdrinking and overdrugging have firm
roots in this human behavioral reality.

White, Bates and Johnson in "Learning to
Drink: Familial, Peer and Media Influences"
(Pittman and Roman 1991) report how
important peer and family influences are for
the young in the society to learn responsible
drinking. The "Just Say No" until twenty-one
policy fails youngsters during their teens
when they are learning all kinds of
self-control measures. The authors state:

> *Drinking alcoholic beverages, like
> other acquired human behaviors, is
> learned and usually performed in a
> social context. There are many
> socially acceptable reasons and
> occasions for alcohol use, many
> social rewards for drinking, and
> many role models of drinking be-
> haviors. These factors have*

> *resulted in the integration of a wide*
> *variety of drinking practices.*

Through all these centuries and in all recorded cultures, alcoholic beverages have been both staple foods and social drinks (Katz 1986). Alcohol remains a basic source of food energy for hundreds of millions across the globe. Ancient Egyptian workers survived comfortably on a diet consisting mainly of bread, beer and onions. Low-alcohol beer was produced in nearly every domicile by soaking sugar-rich bread pieces in water vessels invoking airborne yeast fermentations.

The ancient Greeks, Egyptians, and Sumerians venerated special gods of wine and beer. The same alcohol-fostering deities represented human fertility, the very principle of life itself. Christianity and Judaism both employ wine as the symbols of human redemption, representing for the Christian the very blood of the Creator and Savior.

America the ambivalent

The root of the "drinking problem" in our nation is ambivalence. Persistent, persuasive and petulant ambivalence about whether to drink, when to drink, and how much to drink.

Sociologist Joseph Gusfield discusses our pesky ambivalence (Douglas 1987):

> *But there are deeper meanings to the use of alcohol in American life that stem from its character as a source of conflict and ambivalence in American life . . . The very derogation of drinking among large segments of American society creates its meaning as a quasi-subterranean behavior when practiced in those segments.*

In other words, making a "big deal" about the "drinking problem" is correct political/religious thinking for some segments of society. But these groups are a minority.

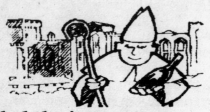

Alcohol the integrator

In Europe's Dark Ages, when the Church assumed both civil and religious authority, monks developed and refined the science of agriculture and the art of wine and beer production and, eventually, became experts in the distillation of spirits. Through all recorded history, drinking has been a common thread in society. Alcohol menstruums serve in medicine and therapy.

Our own Pilgrims brought generous stores of beer with them to sustain them on the perilous passage to the New World. Among their very first tasks, our forefathers provided for beer and wine production. Puritan Increase Mather described drinking as "this good creature of God" praising its sustaining qualities while condemning its abuse. Through all history, though hedged-in by rules and social constraints, alcoholic beverages have had important dietary and social roles (Heath 1987).

Alcohol the disintegrator

Though uplifting, inspiring, and integrative when used in moderation, alcohol has been universally devastating in abuse. At times it has been grossly destructive of human health and of the common good of entire societies. The waning years of the Roman society and the disreputable gin era in early seventeenth century England are frightful examples.

The tendency to excess makes civil alcohol controls absolutely mandatory. The first

written legal code of mankind, decreed by
Hammurabi in ancient Assyria, devoted more
rules to the control of alcohol than to any
other subject. Hammurabi's laws were so
severe that an innkeeper could lose a limb for
overserving. Every society since Hammurabi
has faced similar problems. Those cultures
with the fewest drinking problems introduce
alcohol early in life and associate it with food.
A wide ranging compilation of
anthropological cross-cultural studies
(Marshall 1979) found:

> *When alcoholic beverages are*
> *defined culturally as a food and / or*
> *medicine, drunkenness seldom is*
> *disruptive.*

Aside from the world of Islam and a few
scattered sects which abstain because of
religious admonitions, societal prohibitions
have failed (Heath 1987).

Preoccupation with problems

Anthropologists speculate that one cause of
our national ambivalence about drinking is
our inordinate emphasis on the pathology of
alcoholism and its abuse (Heath 1987).

> *Researchers, clinicians, and others*
> *who pay attention to alcoholic*

> *beverages in those contexts focus*
> *their attention almost exclusively*
> *on pathological outcomes of drink-*
> *ing, whether in terms of economic*
> *cost, physical or mental disability,*
> *social disruption, or in other terms*
> *. . . Similarly, the importance of*
> *drinking as "normal"'behavior (and*
> *not necessarily "deviant") behavior*
> *has rarely been recognized in other*
> *disciplines.*

Another contributing factor emphasized
by researchers is the disintegration of social
systems in our large metropolitan cities
(Marshall 1979).

> *Solitary, addictive, pathological*
> *drinking behavior does not occur to*
> *any significant extent in small-*
> *scale, traditional, pre-industrial*
> *societies. Such behavior appears to*
> *be a concomitant of complex,*
> *modern, industrialized societies.*

Yet, most drinking in our country is normal
and non-deviant. About two-thirds of
American adults drink alcoholic beverages
today (*Bottom Line* 1987). A minority of from
five to ten percent of that number drinks, at
least periodically, to excess. Over
ninety-percent of those who choose to imbibe

can be classified as light to moderate drinkers
(DHHS Report 1987). Much of our
ambivalence can be blamed on public
policymakers. Since the government chooses
to trumpet alcohol's problems and to ignore
it's benefits, many consumers remain
confused and uncertain. In this negative
atmosphere, politicians take the easy-out by
supporting stiffer control measures.

Even though a great many choose to
abstain—more than any other industrialized
nation—the United States is decidedly a wet
nation. Public polls evidence this continuing
intent (Linsky 1986 and Gallup 1988) among
the majority to remain wet. The "problem" is
that for nearly two centuries the minority of
anti-drinking activists has dominated the
public agenda. In government affairs,
drinking is treated only as a tolerable evil.

This public antipathy contrasts with
practices in many European nations which
have, not surprisingly, significantly less
abuse problems. In Europe, drinking is an
accepted and generally acclaimed practice.
Wine, beer and spirits are both food and drink
(Mendelson 1985). In our nation, any
scientific statement concerning the health
values or the propriety of drinking is met with
public doubt and social hostility.

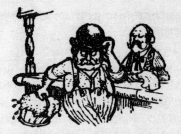

Moderates recognize benefits

Moderate drinkers know that their drinking habits are not harmful. What they lack are official sources of information on the specific benefits from a health viewpoint. An objective evaluation of the research literature muxt become part of the larger debate on the role of alcohol in modern society.

In the last decade, the control debate has intensified and taken on new and controversial dimensions, particularly with the emergence of drunk-driving and drug abuse advocacy groups such as Mothers Against Drunk Driving (*Bottom Line* 1987, Chalke 1981, Franke 1987, Gunby 1987, Gusfield 1981) and the massive government funding of the War on Drugs. Anti-alcohol coalitions include a wide range of civic and social organizations such as the National Council on Alcoholism, the National Institute on Alcohol Abuse and Alcoholism, the American Public Health Association and the Center for Science in the Public Interest, the

Parent Teachers Association and many state medical societies.

Similar confederations of activists have been formed in nations from Australia to England. They use a common language and seek nearly identical political goals which include vastly increased alcohol taxes, the curtailment or total elimination of liquor advertising and many normal sales promotion practices, the raising of the minimum legal drinking age, a lessening of retail availability and the association of drinking with illicit street drugs.

This is known as the Control of Availability agenda. The rules and regulations make alcohol hard to get and prohibitively costly with the hope that abusers will abuse less.

These are mostly governmental policies desgined to discourage any alcohol intake (American Medical Association 1968, Bowen 1987). This incessant negative public advocacy has led many light and moderate consumers to question their customary drinking habits. Moderates are beginning to doubt the values and the propriety of drinking. Recent attitude surveys of non-drinkers (Ellison 1990) reveal that 58 percent believed there were no benefits in drinking and 55 percent felt it bad for one's health. Sadly, the government propaganda is working well.

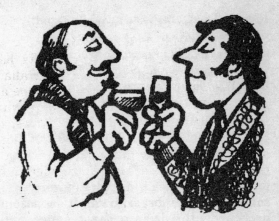

The medical muzzle

The positive data is out there but the coalition of an overcautious government and a highly vocal private advocacy make it difficult for doctors and other health authorities to endorse moderate drinking— or even to be positive about the practice.

Doctors are sitting ducks for lawsuits, as are the producers of wine, beer and spirits. In a penetrating analysis of the crisis in tort law in our society titled *Liability: The Legal Revolution and its Consequences,* Huber argues (Huber 1988) that the main problem lies in getting the lawyer out of the mix so *fearless* communication can once again occur. Huber writes:

> *The answer surely cannot be to
> banish the technology itself, for
> that would prevent us from saving
> many lives and much suffering. . . .
> With lawyers not so prominent in
> the picture, doctor and patient can
> find ways to recognize their
> common interests, as can employer
> and employee.*

This book is a limited answer to this communication breakdown. It is possible, without entering into the broader public debate about the propriety of drinking, or the nature and extent of its civil controls, to define the limits of moderate, healthful drinking from the available science and research.

Before addressing the medical findings, there follows discussions on drinking terms and on how much is too much.

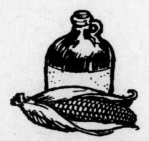

Chapter 5

Definitions

Here are definitions of the common terms used in the scientific literature on alcohol and health. Those who wish to drink in a responsible manner should be familiar with this basic terminology.

Absolute alcohol. Scientists generally convert the various drinks into the actual grams of ethanol (ethyl alcohol) consumed. There are 28 grams in each fluid ounce of pure or absolute alcohol. If a person reports the average of 4 drinks consumed per day it means approximately 56 grams of absolute alcohol.

Wines, beers and spirits contain varying
amounts of ethanol. Beer, as example,
normally contains between 3.5 and 4 percent
absolute alcohol (by weight) mingled into 11
to 12 ounces of water and other constituents.
An eleven ounce bottle of beer, then, contains
about half an ounce of absolute alcohol.

Spirituous liquors have a much higher
ethanol concentration. An 80 proof rum
contains 40 percent ethanol compared to the
4 percent for beer. Since we pour about an
ounce for our favorite drinks we actually
consume slightly under a half ounce of
absolute alcohol in every drink. With wine
there is no doubt. The volume of alcohol in the
bottle is clearly marked on the label. If your
wine glass contains 6 ounces of a wine that is
12 percent by volume, the glass contains .72
percent of an ounce of absolute alcohol.

This is what the recent "equivalency"
campaign of the distillers was all about.
Distillers point out that a bottle of beer, a one
ounce cocktail and a five ounce glass of wine
contain identical amounts of absolute alcohol.
A moderate drinker, therefore, must
understand and calculate the amounts of
absolute alcohol contained in various drinks
in order to maintain a safe level of intake. The
amounts of alcohol used in various drinks are
found in cocktail and mixed drink manuals. It
is my hope that all alcohol-containing

beverages will someday be clearly identified
by *volume* as is the case now with wine.

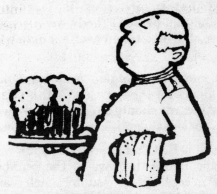

Beer and malt beverages. These are
fermented beverages from cereal grains
which have been malted (germinated) to
convert the grain starch into fermentable
maltose sugar. The maltose ferments into
ethyl alcohol and carbon dioxide just like
wine. *Malt liquors* in the United States are a
class of beers which contain higher absolute
alcohol levels. Popular malt beverage styles
include ale, bock, lager, pilsner and wheat
(weiss) beers.

Blood alcohol content. Blood alcohol
content (BAC or BAL) is a measurement of
the absolute alcohol circulating in a person's
bloodstream after drinking. Many BAC
pocket cards are available. The Washington
State Liquor Control Board has distributed

the Rutgers card for years in its state stores. The Rutgers card depicts the approximate alcohol concentrations in eight weight categories. It provides BAC readings according to a person's body weight and the number of drinks taken over a single hour of time.

You can surely blame American alcohol ambivalence for the spare use of this effective tool. BAC cards should be distributed through all driver licensing outlets in the nation.

To use a BAC card, you find your weight and look across the card to the number of drinks necessary for you to reach various levels of BAC up to legal intoxication. As example, a 100 pound person will become legally intoxicated after consuming the fourth average drink (containing approximately one-half ounce of absolute alcohol each) within a single hour. The same person spacing three of those drinks over a two hour party will remain in control of his faculties and never become legally intoxicated.

While .10 BAC represents legal intoxication in most states, it is critical to understand that a person begins to lose some physical control and manual dexterity after the first drink. Intoxication is progressive from the first appearance of ethanol in the bloodstream. For this reason, the Washington card and most other BAC cards also depict an "impaired zone" beginning at .05 BAC in which driving or other life-threatening or dangerous activities such as swimming are inadvisable.

However many mixed drinks—a manhattan or a malt liquor—may contain up to a full ounce of absolute alcohol. This is double the standard drink implied on the BAC card. BAC cards provide *averages only* and they do not account for emotional states of mind, experience in drinking or the physical differences among men and women drinkers.

Many other factors come into play. The very young or new drinkers of any are less tolerant and unused to alcohol's intoxicative effects. Disturbed or distressed individuals, or those eating large meals, will experience different rates of absorption of alcohol. Even with these variables, the BAC cards can provide prudent guidelines for the responsible drinker.

Cardiovascular and heart disease terms. Since much of the current interest involving alcohol and health has to do with heart and cardiovascular diseases (CVD), a few common medical terms will be helpful in interpreting reports in this book and casual articles in the media.

According to the American Heart Association, nearly 65 million Americans have heart or blood vessel disease of some sort and 991,300 individuals died of these causes in 1985. According to the AHA, nearly one-third of our population have one form or another of heart vessel impairment.

High density lipoprotein (HDL) and low density lipoprotein (LDL) are two important cholesterol components in the blood. HDL is known as the *good form of cholesterol* because it helps cleanse the arteries of the constricting plaques formed in part by the presence of LDL, *the bad cholesterol.*

Myocardial infarction (MI) means a heart attack. Morbidity means disease and mortality means death. In many clinical and epidemiological studies, moderate alcohol intake has been associated with better heart morbidity or health (Breslow 1980, Camargo 1984, Castelli 1984, Ferrence 1986, Freidman 1983, Gill 1986, Haskell 1984, Klatsky 1981, Moore 1986, and Stamler 1985).

There is some debate over the relevance of these findings (Knupfer 1987) but general agreement (Klatsky 1985, Lieber 1984 and

Richman 1984) that moderate drinking is a component in life-styles conducive to heart health. Discussing what is now called the French Paradox, Ellison (Ellison 1990) finds wine as a possible explanation why Frenchmen have lower rates of CVD despite relatively high intake of fat and high levels of smoking.

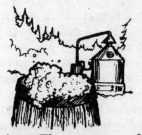

Distillation. The process of vaporizing beer, wine or other alcohol mashes in a heating device is distillation. The vessel boils off portions of the ethyl alcohol and other constituents from the beer or wine. Since alcohol vaporizes at a much lower temperature than water, the first steam contains high amounts of ethanol and chemicals called congeners. When cooled, this steam liquifies and forms the spirituous beverage.

The various grains and fruits used to ferment the alcohol mash and the level at which the steam is taken from the still determine the tastes of the *proof* or alcohol content of the original spirit. The differences in taste for various spirits originates in the percentage of congeners carried over from the mash.

Bourbon, as example, is produced from a mash of corn with lesser amounts of barley and rye. Smoke-treated barley is used to create the distinctive aromas and tastes in the single malt scotch. Blended scotch includes tempering quantities of lighter corn whiskey. Tequila is distilled from a mash fermented from the highly aromatic maguey plant. If all the congeners or impurities are boiled away, the resulting alcohol has little flavor and is called neutral spirits. When neutral spirits are further purified through charcoal, they may be called vodkas.

Drinking levels. Since our nation includes many diverse cultures and heritages, each with a distinctive approach to drinking, there are inevitable differences about what constitutes moderation in drinking. Here are some sensible drinking standards which appeared in the *Second Special Report to Congress on Alcohol and Health* published by the National Institute on Alcohol Abuse and Alcoholism. These standards are non-judgmental. They can include a wide range of drinking habits including the German and Italian daily drinking of generous amounts of wine and beer.

> **Moderate Occasional.** *Persons*
> *who drink any form of alcohol but*
> *only in small amounts at any one*
> *time, never enough to become*
> *intoxicated, and less frequent*
> *than daily.*
> **Moderate Steady.** *Same as*
> *for Moderate Occasional, except*
> *daily.*
> **Heavy Occasional.** *Persons*
> *who get drunk occasionally, with*
> *periods of either abstinence or*
> *moderate drinking.*
> **Heavy.** *Persons who get drunk*
> *regularly and frequently.*

Fermentation. This is the natural process in which a source of sugar is catalyzed by yeast enzymes yielding equal parts of ethyl alcohol and carbon dioxide. All alcoholic beverages derive their alcohols from natural fermentation.

Moderate drinking. Moderate drinking is best defined as that which maintains sobriety and control of faculties so as to avoid danger to self and others. The World Health Organization (WHO) has suggested the upper limits of moderate drinking at 60 grams a day and/or less than the amount required to reach the .10 BAC level of intoxication (Babor 1987).

Social drinking is defined by World Health Organization as that which conforms with local norms and expectations. WHO has suggested an upper limit of moderate drinking of no more than 60 grams (four drinks) of absolute alcohol daily and/or less than an amount required to reach a .10 BAC which is intoxication (Babor 1987).

In large nations, like the United States, drinking norms vary widely in regions and among ethnic and social groupings. In our pluralistic society the only sensible norm for drinking is that which advises individuals not to drink to excess. That is, drinking should be paced so that the individual remains at or below the .05 BAC and in control of faculties at all times. It is irrational, laughable policy at NIAAA that two drinks a day constitutes heavy drinking.

For some, a drink once a week with friends or associates constitutes moderate drinking. For others, remaining under the .05 BAC whenever drinking may be responsible behavior. Moderation is as much a frame of mind as a scientific measurement. Though more common sense than science, the "ABC's of Drinking & Driving" published by Mothers Against Drunk Driving suggests six social performance standards which combine to assure moderation whatever the drinking conditions. They are:

> 1. ***EAT FIRST.*** *Food slows the rate of alcohol absorption.*
> 2. ***DRINK SLOWLY.*** *Space your drinks to avoid rapid intoxication.*
> 3. **KNOW WHAT'S BEING DRUNK** *It is impossible to compute BAC levels without a knowledge of the absolute alcohol levels of each drink.*
> 4. **SET A LIMIT.** *Plan the maximum number of drinks for any occasion and stick to the decision.*
> 5. **STOP IN TIME.** *Allow the body to work your BAC down to safe levels before driving or engaging in other demanding activities.*
> 6. **BE HONEST.** *These are common sense recommendations which provide a framework for moderate intake.*

Proof. Under a completely inane federal regulation, spirituous liquors are measured in terms of *proof.* Proof is a hangover from the Middle Ages. Proof is exactly double the actual absolute alcohol content. An 80 proof brandy contains 40 percent alcohol by volume. A 34 proof peppermint schnapps contains 17 percent absolute alcohol. Wine labels show the exact volumetric measurement of ethanol. Why not switch to volume and dump proof?

Spirits. Spirituous liquors are distilled from wine, beer or other alcoholic mash and sold following a dilution with distilled water at levels ranging from 80 to 151 proof. Included are whisky, gin, vodka, rum, schnapps, liqueurs, and pre-mixed cocktails including spirituous beverages.

Standard drink. This is a research or control concept. In the real world, there is no such thing as a standard drink. Only beer is sold regularly in a single drink container, though both wine and spirits have single bottle servings.

Many prevention and alcohol control manuals refer to a standard drink as one which contains one-half ounce of absolute alcohol. Bars vary their pours from under an ounce to an ounce and a half. Home poured drinks often reach two ounces. Wines vary in alcohol content from 9 percent in a German liebfraumilch to 14 percent in a robust

California zinfandel table wine and from 5 to 8 ounces in glass servings..

Beer varies in alcohol from around 2 percent in low alcohol (LA) styles to nearly 6 percent in malt liquors. To complicate this swamp of confusion, beer is measured by the feds by the *weight* of alcohol rather than volume—the only beverage so measured. Alcohol weight is close to volume, but not identical to it.

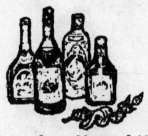

Spirits range from 80 proof (40 percent alcohol) to 151 proof in some rums. Some mixed drinks such as a manhattan, rob roy or Long Island Iced Tea call for as much as a full ounce of absolute alcohol from various spirit combinations.

The absolute alcohol in single serving containers varies widely. If a wine cooler lists 5 percent alcohol by volume there is .60% of an ounce in the 12 ounce bottle. That is exactly the same amount contained in a 6 percent malt liquor but both are less than the .80% of an ounce in a martini which contains two ounces of 80 proof gin. One ounce of 17 percent schnapps has only .17 percent of an ounce of absolute alcohol.

With such a variety of sources and amounts of absolute alcohol in popular beverages today, drinkers should become knowledgeable about the alcohol content of the drinks they choose.

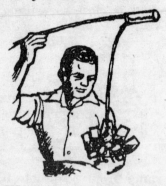

Wine. Wines form the third great family of alcoholic beverages and they are naturally fermented from a fruit mash. Naturally fermented still or table wines range from 9 to 14 percent alcohol. The level depends upon the amount of sugar in the grapes and the length of the fermentation period.

Sparkling wines are produced through the secondary fermentation of still wines. The carbon dioxide is retained in the bottle from that secondary ferment to create the universally pleasing effervescence.

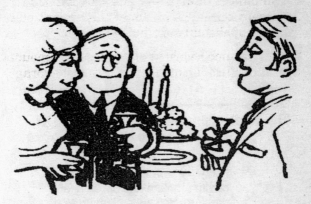

Aperitif and dessert wines. These wines generally have higher alcohol levels because of the addition of varying amounts of brandy (distilled wine). Aperitif (before eating) and dessert (after eating wines) are served in small glasses and are designed to either stimulate the appetite or to finish off a gracious meal.

The alcohol concentrations in specialty wines range from 16 to 20 percent by volume orroughly double the alcohol in table wines. The brandy used to fortify dessert wines is produced by distilling an already fermented table wine.

It's been written . . .

Heavy alcohol use is both a health problem and public health problem. However, blaming alcohol as the culprit in every malady in which it is found frequently has the effect of diminishing other possible explanations.

David R. Ruby, "The Adult Children of Alcoholics Movement" in Society, Culture and Drinking Patterns Reexamined, Pittman and White, Rutgers Center of Alcohol Studies, 1991

Chapter 6

Upper Limits of Consumption

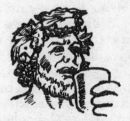

People who choose to drink need to know the levels at which they endanger physical and psychological well-being. They don't need scare campaigns about addiction and drugs.

One thing is a certainty. Current government guidelines for drinking are arbitrary and unscientific, In fact, nearly all decisions at Health and Human Services about drinking are colored by political—not scientific—considerations. HHS now advises an upper limit of two drinks per day for men and a single libation for women. These "two and one" limits ignore variables in body size, gender, age, drinking experience, the social conditions in which the drinking occurs, cultural and ethnic heritages, the known science on drinking and social realities. In sum, HHS recommendations on drinking are unscientific and politically motivated.

Drinking dangers well known

The problems of heavy drinking are well publicized. Media awareness campaigns in cooperation with public safety and alcoholism agencies have been very effective in recent years using what is called the "systems approach." As a nation, we can be proud of this cooperative effort particularly in the area of drunken driving. The public is coming to understand that overdrinking stems from very complex human motivations.

An unfortunate, but inevitable, byproduct of the "systems approach" is the sensational media coverage of drinking problems. Quite naturally, the media thrives on gore and titillation, especially when prominent figures are involved in the incidents.

We are deluged by books, magazine articles, movies and television dramas showing the ill effects of abuse and binge drinking (Eckhard 1981, Ferrence 1986 and Knupfer 1987). The reports of benefits are sporadic and not nearly so interesting as the serious automobile wreck or shots of an intoxicated offender. In this milieu, there remains a high level of confusion in the public mind about drinking and health (Chalke 1981, Education Commission of the States 1980, Gastineau 1979, Gordon 1987, Heath 1987 and Lieber 1984). In comparison to other nations, we dwell inordinately on the problems and misfortunes.

What the science really says

In 1988, the Gallup organization reported a mere 17 percent in the nation favoring a return to prohibition, the lowest number since this question was first asked by Gallup pollsters in the 1930s. Though nearly one-third of the population abstains, less than twenty percent believe the prohibitions work.

Another Gallup poll in 1987 reported that over eighty percent of respondents support alcohol health warnings. Citizens apparently want to continue drinking even though they have nagging doubts as to the health factors.

I mention these conflicting polls before presenting the existing science on the upper limits of drinking to show the confusion among drinkers and nondrinkers alike. We must begin to resolve these questions and uncertainties about drinking and health in order to implement rational control policies.

I use the upper limit for drinking taken from a 1981 survey of the medical literature published in the *Johns Hopkins Medical Journal* titled "The Beneficial Side of Moderate Alcohol Use" (Turner 1981). I have not found any challenge to either the scholarship or the findings set forth in this elaborate study. I have published excerpts from it twice in the *Moderation Reader*.

Consequently, I was shocked to find in a recently published analysis that NIAAA characterize this study as "old research." This language was used by NIAAA in a letter to Alcohol, Tobacco and Firearms commenting on the impact of alcohol warning labels. This cavalier dismissal of a ten year old research survey is beyond my understanding. Does NIAAA believe that science—like old soldiers—is supposed to simply fade away.

The government deliberately ignores the good news about drinking. The growing awareness of the heart health benefits of moderate drinking is not due to government communication but to programs like the "French Paradox" on *60 Minutes*. And to the media coverage of the increasing numbers of positive studies (American Heart Association 1987, Camargo 1985, Friedman 1983, Gordon 1983, Haskel 1984 and Moore 1986). The recognition of lowered risk of high blood pressure and stroke in moderate drinking is similarly cumulative (American Heart Association 1987, Glieberman 1986, and

Donahue 1986). The healthy lifestyles of moderate drinkers are also found abundantly (Brewslow 1980, Health 1987, Klatsky 1981 and Lieber 1984).

The Turner study cites dozens of these studies in concluding its upper limit of 80 grams per day, one third higher than the WHO's 60 gram recommendation. The difference is that Turner looked to the medical literature for evidences of organic damage. The WHO recommendation is based on political/social objectives, not the extant research.

In considering this upper limit, it is very important to distinguish between harmless levels and *recommended* levels. An 80 gram intake is approximately five average drinks. At no point does Turner's recommend that anyone drink at that relatively high level. The researchers simply found no organic harm from any single day's consumption at 80 grams. It is important to note that the NIAAA calls five or more drinks harmful "binge drinking." This is the critical difference between the science and politics of drinking.

Women should drink less

One thing all researchers agree on—and common sense tells us—is that women should drink less. This is one area in which the sexes

are unequal. One reason is body size. Women
are generally smaller than men. Since alcohol
circulates in the bloodstream, larger blood
systems accomodate more alcohol. No matter
the body size, one hour is required for a
healthy liver to oxidize each and every drink.
In the elimination rate, men and women are
equal. But, since women are smaller bodied,
they will have higher BACs during this
process if they toss down drinks one-for-one
with men.

Christopher Gilson has written extensively
about women and drinking. "Although for
years BAC charts have been in wide use . . .
it is known that pound for pound of body
weight, women reach higher peaks than men
from the same quantity of alcohol (Gilson
1989)." Gilson cites more recent research in
Oklahoma and Britain (Gilson 1991)that
"found that women reached about 1.4 times
the (alcohol) peaks for men from the same
quantities of alcohol per pound of body
weight."

Another factor has to do with body fat.
Women and older persons, on average, have a
greater percentage of body fat and less bodily
fluids. A new line of research (Steinbrook
1990) shows "that women appear to have
significantly lower amounts of stomach
enzymes" than men. These are the enzymes
that break down alcohol.

Women should also be aware of growing evidence of a higher risk of liver damage probably because of the longer periods of exposure in the bloodstream (Norton 1987).

All of these factors counsel a more conservative drinking regimen for women but hardly the "one-a-day" recommended by HHS.

Daily drinking

No long-term adverse health effects have been identified from moderate daily drinking. The reverse of that coin is that dozens of long-term *health benefits have been found* in daily drinking.

Many epidemiological surveys associate either frequent and periodic drinking or light daily consumption with positive health effects, most notably decreased risk of coronary heart disease and greater longevity (Klatsky 1981). It is uncertain whether regularity in drinking creates or merely contributes to these positive health effects.

However, it is known that when a person stops regular daily drinking, there are losses in protective effects which place that individual at greater risk such as a reduction in the levels of high density lipoprotein (Camargo 1985). In pursuing an overall reduction in per capita drinking, government

health officials ignore this *increased* danger
in abstinence and place the entire drinking
population at greater risk. Hardly a public
health service.

Daily drinking is not harmful in itself. In a
series of commentaries on drinking in a recent
British Journal of Addiction titled "Drinking
Sensible," one contributor stated that as
many as 96.6 percent of individuals who drink
within the suggested upper limits experience
no adverse effects from alcohol (Kendell
1987).

Dr. Elizabeth Whelan, director of the
American Council on Science and Health has
written extensively about this distinction
(Whelan 1991). She concludes:

> *Now for the answer you've been
> waiting for. From all the scientific
> literature, it appears that one-and-
> a-quarter to two-and-a-half ounces
> of absolute alcohol a day carry few,
> if any, health risks and may be
> beneficial. That's about two-and-a-
> half to five drinks as defined
> above—the equivalent of two of the
> little bottles of liquor sold on the
> airlines.*

For light to moderate daily drinkers, the
risks are minimal and the benefits both

tangible and numerous. We should not jeopardize these advantages in a mistaken prohibitionary fervor.

Who should not drink

Some people should never drink. Every drinker of every age or sex should use prudence and caution in their drinking habits. Recovering alcoholics should abstain according to the current consensus in the medical community (Mendelson 1985, Public Policy on Alcohol Problems 1984, Turner 1984 and Turner 1987).

Anyone planning to drive an automobile, to engage in heavy work or sports, or to operate life-threatening machinery shortly after drinking should exercise particular caution and remain well below the .05 BAC zone.

Individuals with histories of adverse physical or mental reactions to drinking and those warned against drinking by their physicians should not indulge at any time. Many common, over-the-counter medications either contain alcohol or act synergistically with alcohol expanding its intoxicating effects. Consumers should always consult medical authority when in doubt about their drinking.

Finally, even light to moderate drinkers should be aware that overdrinking often is associated with periods of life stress. When things go wrong at work or in a marriage, people tend to overdrink. Wars or major disruptions in social, economic or political affairs often precipitate widespread alcohol abuse among the normally moderate.

Setting calorie limits

Alcohol can be considered a simple food since its chemical reduction within the body releases usable calories. Calories are the reason we eat. People who overdrink often gain weight just as those who overeat.

When an 180 pound man consumes five eleven-ounce beers, he adds 700 calories or about one-third of his total daily caloric requirement. Setting calorie limits is another approach to maintaining moderation in daily drinking. Recommended daily limits for alcohol calories (American Heart Association 1986, Turner 1981) range from ten to twenty percent of the total diet. The American Heart Association recommends an absolute upper daily limit of 15 percent of daily calories.

American drinkers average about 8 percent of their calories from alcohol (Turner 1981). Since these beverages serve both as social drinks and as mealtime beverages, a daily drinker is wise to count both alcohol calories and blood alcohol levels.

Drinking should invoke the same prudent constraints that a person applies to coffee, chocolate or tea intake.

No absolute answers

If you are looking for absolute guidelines on drinking, you will not find them in this book. That is because such absolutes do not exist in either science or culture. This book does not endorse drinking nor does it recommend abstinence but it does reject soundly NIAAA's "two for men and one for women."

Many cultural, physical, financial, ethical, religious and social factors should come into consideration in decisions about drinking. In "Lesson on Drinking: The Italians Do It Best" (Health 1988), there is this definitive quote about the common sense approach:

> *When we talk about Culture, we*
> *refer to attitudes and values as well*
> *as to customs and patterns of be-*
> *havior . . . wholesome attitudes and*
> *customs should be fostered . . . that*
> *assure that drinking continues to*
> *be a pleasant part of life rather*
> *than a mysterious danger.*

It's been written . . .

French men, as a group, smoke more, exercise less, eat thirty percent more saturated fat in the form of butter, cheese, lard and foie gras, yet have one-third to one-half as many heart attacks as a similar group of American men. French men also drink red wine with their lunch and dinner, up to ten times as much as American men. This so-called "French Paradox" of increased heart health along with "bad" health habits, lead many investigators to wonder if the red wine in the diet provides a protective element to the coronary vessels.

Paul Scholten, M.D., San Francisco wine journalist

Part III

The

Good

News

Chapter 7

The physiology of drinking

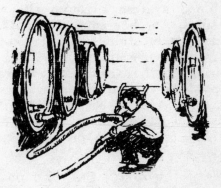

Not only is alcohol abundant in nature, but it is produced and eliminated regularly and naturally within every human body. Alcohol is a natural bodily fluid.

Ethyl alcohol is not foreign to human physiology. Up to one ounce is produced daily in humans by bacterial breakdown of starches and sugars. Small amounts of alcohol are consumed in fruit juices and medicines. So, while there are many non-drinkers, there are no real abstainers. Man-made alcohol is oxidized in the liver in the same manner as that intentionally consumed. Here's how the metabolizing process works.

As we consume licensed beverages, very small portions of the alcohols in them pass into the bloodstream through the mouth and the stomach walls. Most of the alcohol enters the blood system through the small intestines. Another small percentage is eliminated in breathing and by the kidneys. But over 90 percent of the alcohol is metabolized by the liver. Since alcohol cannot be deposited in human cells in the manner of other drugs, the alcohol circulates in the bloodstream until dehydrogenase enzymes in the liver reduce it to water and carbon dioxide.

One of the distinctive and positive attributes of alcohol is the fact that it cannot lodge in organs and tissues as do, for instance, harmful chemicals from marijuana and cocaine. The body initiates the process of elimination of alcohol immediately after assimilation. A healthy liver oxidizes about one drink each hour (American Medical Association 1968) but this process is not absolute (Goldstein 1983):

> *The rate at which ethanol*
> *disappears from the blood varies*
> *widely among individuals. A*

> *general rule is useful, even if crude.*
> *For this purpose, one can use the*
> *figure of 10 ml of absolute alcohol*
> *per hour for an average-size man.*
> *Small people, women, and*
> *teenagers may be expected to*
> *eliminate ethanol more slowly, in*
> *general.*

The body uses the newly released energy immediately. All traces of ethanol in each drink are therefore dissipated within an hour of consumption. Ethanol alcohol, then, enters and leaves the body within an hour leaving no physical or mental impairments. However, many individuals in social sessions drink more than a single drink an hour. They must remember that the ethanol will circulate in the blood—with its intoxicating properties affecting the brain—until the liver eventually catches up at the rate of one drink per hour. The key, then, is to maintain a *sober rate* of drinking.

Food retards intoxication

Any ethanol in the bloodstream acts as a depressant on the central nervous system. But in moderate amounts, alcohol relaxes a human through its physiological impacts—dilating blood vessels, lowering blood pressure and heightening physical senses (Olsen 1985). These physical reactions combine to produce light intoxication and euphoria, the sense of well-being which is the very object of drinking.

Food in the stomach, particularly fats and proteins, retards alcohol absorption by slowing the emptying of the gut. Food may slow alcohol absorption by as much as 50 percent contributing to lower overall peak concentrations. For the same amount of drinks consumed, scientists have found lower BACs from alcohol consumed with a full meal and up to two hours after. The trick is never to consume alcohol without some form of food.

At a BAC of .05 percent, reaction-time is slightly impaired but the drinker is generally in charge of his or her faculties. At .08 to 1.0 BAC levels, there is a marked loss of motor control, speech is blurred and prudent judgment is invalidated. At .20 BAC, emotional and physical instability are apparent. At .40 BAC, the body becomes comatose, the dead-drunk stage which protects the human from further drinking until the life-threatening levels of alcohol are eliminated. A BAC of .50 can result in death.

Like riding in an automobile, drinking can be dangerous. But also like the automobile, when used correctly, drinking adds to the general well being of the individual and benefits society at large.

Chapter 8

Drinking and the heart

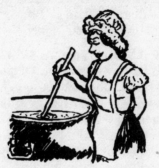

The French paradox is but the tip of the health iceberg. There is a really massive amount of positive research about drinking and the heart. Heart disease is the American nemesis, the cause of nearly half of our premature morbidity and mortality. So the real paradox is that so few Americans know the good news about drinking.

Research reports that moderate drinking lowers the risk of heart attacks. The paradox is that so few Americans are made aware of this factor by health authorities.

The American Heart Association estimates that nearly 65 million people have one or more forms of heart or blood vessel disease

(American Heart Association 1988). This menacing roster includes heart attacks, stroke, high blood pressure, rheumatic fever, atherosclerosis and congenital heart conditions. In 1900, 15 percent of deaths were from heart disease. The toll had risen to 50 percent by 1967 (Ellison 1990).

Start with the certainty that *heavy drinking is bad for the heart.* Of this, there is no medical question. Excessive intake has been causally linked to cardiomyopathy, hypertension and increased risk of stroke (*Alcohol Report* 1987, Eckhard 1981 and Knupfer 1987). However, as early as 1904, light to moderate drinking was linked to a decrease of the risk of heart disease (Mendelson 1985). One study of 18 developed countries found (Leger 1979):

> *The principal finding is a strong
> and specific negative association
> between ischemic heart disease
> deaths and alcohol consumption
> wholly attributable to wine
> consumption.*

Another paper surveyed over 160 alcohol and heart studies involving more than 100,000 individuals over a span of sixty years (Moore 1986). These authors found a pattern in which the incidence of both coronary artery

disease and cardiovascular mortality
decreased with increasing levels of
consumption up to 4 to 5 drinks daily:

> *A rich and diverse literature*
> *documents the association between*
> *alcohol consumption and coronary*
> *artery disease using a variety of*
> *methods. . . The consistency,*
> *strength, specificity, dose-response,*
> *and independence of the associa-*
> *tion between moderate alcohol*
> *consumption and CAD implies*
> *a causal relationship.*

Another convincing study inventoried
drinking and other factors in the small town
of Framingham, Massachusetts for over
twenty-five years. In this continuing study,
cardiovascular disease has been found to be
inversely related to regular drinking (Gordon
1983). In Framingham, regular drinkers have
less heart trouble.

The beat goes on

I could rest my case for moderate drinking
and heart health right here. Researchers
don't use the word *causal* casually. But the
healthy beat goes on.

Researchers favor "prospective" studies because many variables can be built into the studies in advance. A spate of prospective studies favor light to moderate drinking.

Dr. Eric Rimm and colleagues at Harvard University studied 51,529 male professionals adjusting for coronary risk factors including dietary intake of cholesterol, fat, fiber and alcohol (Rimm 1991). The authors found that men who drank, on average, three to four days per week had a lower risk of heart disease than men who drank less than one day each week. They concluded that the "inverse association between alcohol intake and the risk of coronary disease is causal."

Another study looked for the relationship of drinking and mortality from all causes. (Lazarus 1991) The subjects included 2225 women and 1835 men over the age of 35. The study encompassed ten years. They found that, among the men, long-term abstainers were at increased risk of death from all causes, though not significantly. Another interesting finding was that women who stopped drinking were at *significantly higher* risk of death from all causes.

Another recent report (Jackson 1991) studied both men and women and concluded that men who had heart attacks were more likely to have been lifelong abstainers and that "the results support the hypothesis that

light and moderate alcohol consumption
reduces the risk of coronary heart disease."

In the Jackson study, as well as a
continuing series of prospective studies by Dr.
Arthur Klatsky at Oakland's Kaiser
Permanente Hospital (Klatsky 1990), former
drinkers were removed from the non-drinker
sample since they might be suffering some
residual ill effects of drinking. The study
included 129,170 individuals. Klatsky also
eliminated other confounding factors. He
concludes:

> *These data should not be used to*
> *justify heavy drinking . . . Lighter*
> *drinkers (those taking up to 1 to 2*
> *drinks / day) were at the lowest risk*
> *of cardiovascular disease and were*
> *not at higher risk of noncardiovas-*
> *cular death.*

The American Cancer Society
commissioned a study among its membership
(Boffetta and Garfinkel 1990) titled "Alcohol
Drinking and Mortality Among Men Enrolled
in the American Cancer Society Prospective
Study." The project included 18,771 men aged
40-59. The risk for coronary heart disease was
reduced progressively for occasional drinkers,
daily drinkers of one drink and even more
signficantly for those who consumed two

drinks a day. Again, overall mortality was also less for drinkers including deaths from cancer.

Gill and associates (Gill 1991) found a similar reduction in strokes from consumption of 100 grams to 300 grams of ethanol per week. There was a 30 to 50 percent reduction of three kinds of strokes: ischemic, subarachnoid and cerebral. The researchers states:

> *The results suggest that low levels
> of alcohol consumption may have
> some protective effect upon the
> cerebral vasculature, whereas
> heavy consumption predisposes
> to both hemorrhagic and
> non-hemorrhagic stroke.*

Ambivalence prevails

One must wonder why the health community is so hesitant to recognize and publicize the health impact of this common food consumed by over two-thirds of adult Americans. The answer, of course, is ambivalence. There is an endemic preoccupation with the *dangers* of overdrinking. Despite findings which confirmed Rimm and Klatsky that moderate drinkers (up to 2 drinks a day) have less heart disease, Marmot (Marmot 1991) concluded that an increase in the mean level of consumption would increase heavy drinking.

> *The balance of harm and benefit
> does not weigh in favor of making a
> recommendation to the public to
> drink in order to prevent heart
> disease.*

Marmot's conclusion errs in two fundamental ways. First, *informing* drinkers of these benefits while encouraging moderation is not the same as encouraging overconsumption. Drinking and overdrinking stem from different impulses.

Second, the scientific literature demonstrates that per capita drinking has little relationship to abusive drinking. Italians and Spaniards drink four times as much as Americans and have markedly less alcoholism and abuse among old and young.

Marmot's pessimism is personal opinion, tacked onto good science. No undue increase in abusive drinking has been noted in any of these many prospective studies. Why not? Because the majority in our nation is moderate and undoubtedly will remain so. This medical paternalism is unseemly and misleading. Just give us the facts and let our native common sense come into play.

One might even conjecture that if Americans consumed as Italians (only about 65% do compared to 90% of Italians and French), we might have significantly *less* heart disease per capita. Our inability to deal with drinking dispassionately may be sentencing untold numbers of citizens to untimely deaths and physical debilitation.

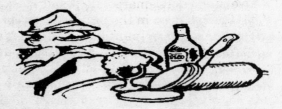

The cholesterols

Many of these heart/alcohol studies report that modest consumption raises the high density lipoprotein (HDL) serum cholesterol concentrations. Cholesterol is one member of a group of compounds called lipids, which cannot dissolve in water. Fats and oils also belong to this family. Since cholesterol cannot dissolve in the blood, a watery medium, it must combine with certain proteins to make it water-soluble.

The cleansing effect of HDL has been confirmed in many papers (Castelli 1984,

Ferrence 1986, Friedman 1983, Gordon 1983, Klatsky 1981, La Porte 1980, Moore 1986, Moore 1988, Stamler 1986 and Turner 1981). HDL cholesterol has the effect of cleaning the tissues and cells of the undesirable low density lipoprotein (LDL) cholesterol deposits. Moore (Moore 1988) writes, "This effect . . . suggests a possible mechanism by which low-dose alcohol may lower the risk of coronary heart disease."

Two studies (Camargo 1985 and Haskell 1984) found a drop in the protective levels of HDL when participants ceased regular drinking. The HDL levels in healthy young males dropped precipitously when daily drinking was curtailed and returned again to satisfactory levels upon resumption of the moderate drinking. Other researchers (La Porte 1980 and St. Leger 1979) reported that nations with higher alcohol per capita levels such as France, Italy, Spain and Portugal had significantly lower rates of cardiovascular morbidity and mortality than low per capita consuming nations such as Finland, Norway and the United States. How can our health officials recommend a lower per capita?

Others describe daily drinking and low-fat dietary habits (La Porte 1980 and McConnell 1987) as conducive to heart health. The McConnells show that while one million Americans are dying from heart diseases, the rate is less than half in wine drinking (and heavy smoking) Italy and Greece. Also, the drinkers have significantly less colon and breast cancer.

Le Paradoxe Francais (Dolnick 1990) concurs with the McConnells by demonstrating that the wine drinking French, "do eat a bit more fat than we do . . . They seem to eat more saturated fat . . . They smoke about as much as we do . . . The French should be having heart attacks everywhere you look. They're not." It's hard to dismiss these observations.

Some disagree with the theory

Critics of these positive findings (Knupfer 1987) suggest that they are flawed because of the presence of former heavy drinkers and the physically ill in the non-drinking segments. To eliminate this distortion, contemporary studies specifically eliminate such individuals (Longnecker 1988 and Richman 1985) and still produce the famed U-curve in which moderate drinkers fare better than non-drinkers. It is apparent that light or daily moderate drinking creates no risks for cardiovascular health and may well, in combination with other life factors, contribute positively to heart health.

A study released by the American Heart
Association (AHA) found that moderate
drinkers had a 49 percent lowered risk of
heart attacks (American Heart Association
1987). The association also cautions women
drinkers to be watchful for an adverse effect
on blood pressure at daily intake levels above
30 to 40 grams. Overall, however, many
studies sponsored by the AHA confirm a
positive relationship between moderate
drinking and heart disease.

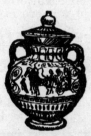

Neodrys ignore health benefits

I am not suggesting that public health
officials should push drinking. Health
professionals should, however, maintain
balance and objectivity when reporting on
serious matters such as drinking and health.

It is apparent that many—perhaps even a
majority—in government and private public
health practice today believe in the WHO goal
of lowering the per capita consumption. But

this conviction ignores a large body of medical research to the contrary.

The health bureaucracy cannot continue to ignore what a drop in consumption *might* mean to moderate drinkers. Could there occur a dramatic *increase* in the incidence of heart disease? Who knows? It's certainly not a public policy to be taken lightly.

In order to emphasize the harmful pathology of alcoholism and abuse, the bureaucracy seeks to stigmatize drinking through an association with the *always harmful* effects of tobacco and illicit street drugs. This policy of downplaying a growing body of research concerning heart health is unconscionable government policy and scandalous public health.

It's been written . . .

If we review the kinds of beverages now used . . by the primitive people of the world, we find that the variety is amazing. A very great number of natural materials were used in their fermentation and brews— berries, fruits, honey,plant saps and, in Central Asia, mare's milk.

Horton, D., *"Alcohol Use in Primitive Societies"* in **Society, Culture and Drinking Patterns, Rexamined,** *Rutgers University 1991*

Chapter 9

Drinking and Stress

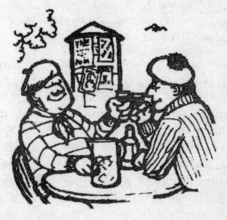

Stress is the most common of human ailments. Alcohol has been a stress reducer (tranquilizer) since before recorded history.

Stress research utilizes sophisticated measurements such as skin conductance and galvanic skin response. Other projects rely upon anecdotal information about the systems and elements used by people to cope with daily stress. Patterns of alcohol use are noted in most stress studies (Turner 1981) and nearly all respondents report lowered emotional tension after moderate drinking.

That expectation is an important precurser to moderate drinking (Robinson 1979):

> *Cultural expectations regulate the emotional consequences of drink. Drinking in one society may regularly release demonstrations of affection; in another it may set off aggressive hostililty.*

Man's oldest stress reducer

Many other cohort and survey studies report a lessening of stress from drinking (Babor 1987, Breslow 1980, Kendell 1987, Licensed Beverage Information Council 1987, Longnecker 1988, Mendelson 1985, Richman 1985, Sarley 1969 and Schaefer 1986). Some deal specifically with drinking and aging (Mishara 1980). Favorable effects of moderate use of alcohol include impacts on sleep patterns, depression, nervous tension, fear and frustration. While excess consumption can stimulate many tension symptoms, there is little controversy that alcohol in moderation has a tranquilizing impact on stressful emotions.

The California Wine Institute published a nifty little physician's handbook about ten years ago (*Wine and Medical Practice* 1979). The introduction contains the following reference to alcohol's role to lessen tension:

> *The oldest of all human ailments*
> *is anxiety, the offspring of fear. It is*
> *still the most universal of all com-*
> *plaints. The widespread desire for*
> *relief from it is attested to by the*
> *use of one million Miltown tablets*
> *in its second year. The caveman*
> *threatened by the saber-toothed*
> *tiger had the same anxiety as the*
> *Wall Street broker in a bear*
> *market. The caveman and the*
> *broker have found in naturally*
> *fermented products a certain*
> *measure of relief.*

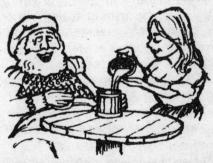

Neoprohibitionists generally ignore the drinking and talking phenomenon, a synergism found uniquely in a tavern or bar. This socializing aspect of drinking is particularly important for singles and for the aging. The contribution of drinking companionship is demonstrated amply in TV's *Cheers*. In his fine book *The Great Good Place* (Oldenburg 1989), Oldenburg writes:

> *The unique potential of the public drinking establishment . . . derives from a fundamental synergism that comes into play wherever alcoholic beverages are part of the culture. . . . The talking / drinking synergism is basic to the pub, tavern, taverna, bistro, saloon, estaminet, osteria— whatever it is called and wherever it is found.*

A good drink and an open ear provides exactly what the drinker seeks. Alcohol is the quintessential chameleon offering to each of us precisely what we seek from it. To the angry and disaffected, drinking infuses wrath. To the contented, a drink opens the mind, relaxes the body and stimulates amiability. Roueche' points to the mind "bemused by alcohol" as one in which:

> *Ideas mount and multiply, affec- tions warm, and memory swells to Proustian proportions. Worries, at a word from reason, bound away.*

Chapter 10

Drinking and aging

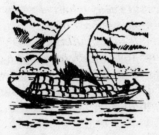

Largely because of its tranquilizing effects, alcohol has been a palliative for older folks for many centuries. There is little doubt that moderate alcohol intake among the elderly improves cognitive performance, reduces worry and aids in sleep (Turner 1981).

One study stressed the contribution of drinking both to the physical and psychological well-being of participants (Mishara 1980 and Kastenbaum 1989). Kastenbaum reports remarkable behavioral changes including continence and the lack of need for physical restraints among patients:

> *... increased morale, reduction in
> worrying, greater ease in falling
> asleep, and improved performance
> on the face-hand test (a basic men-
> tal orientation measure). ... The
> positive changes noted on some
> cognitive tasks were perhaps the
> most impressive results from a
> scientific standpoint.*

Many, if not most, physicians advise a
small daily alcohol regimen to improve the
quality of life with elderly patients. There
seems little evidence that this administration
increases alcohol abuse (Mishara 1980). But
alcohol's effect on longevity is not as certainly
established as its stress-reducing qualities.

Drinking and longevity

However, as in the heart health studies,
researchers find that individuals with levels
of intake up to one ounce of absolute alcohol
(two drinks) daily live longer than those who
abstain completely or consume above this
level (Breslow 1980, Gordon 1987, Klatsky
1981, Linsky 1986, Longnecker 1986,
Mishara 1980, Richman 1985 and Turner
1981).

Two long-term prospective projects
(Breslow 1980 and Klatsky 1981) report

significantly longer life spans among
moderate drinkers.

The lower level of heart disease among
moderate drinkers may contribute to this
apparent increased longevity. Nationwide
health surveys (Longnecker 1988 and
Richman 1985) in the United States and
Canada confirm no specific lessening of
lifespan from moderate daily drinking. From
these reports it is reasonable to assume that
daily drinking becomes a small but important
component in an overall temperate, relaxed
lifestyle which can influence longevity.

One paper confirms the gradual easing of
heavy drinking patterns in the aging (Stall
1987):

> *Probably the most interesting find-*
> *ing to have been replicated in the*
> *alcohol and aging literature is that*
> *a decrease in the prevalence of*
> *heavy, problematical drinking*
> *seems to occur as a concomitant*
> *of the aging process.*

What is important is the knowledge that
reasonable people may drink to a healthy old
age without physical danger—including the
unrealistic fear of developing addictive,
compulsive drinking habits.

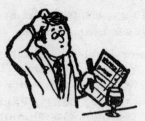

Another recent study (DeLabry 1992) of alcohol consumption and heart disease found that the oldest drinkers had the lowest rate of death from heart disese. The study was carried out at a Veterans' Affairs outpatient facility in Boston. Commentary in the article's conclusion raises the central question of this book—why *fear of overdrinking* is dominating public policy:

> *Copious evidence shows that heavy drinking is harmful to health. On the other hand, a growing body of evidence indicates that moderate drinking may have long term beneficial health effects. Thus, public perception of alcohol has come under the influence of two conflicting trends.*
>
> *One segment of the public health community, influenced by anticipated difficulty in teaching controlled-drinking practices in some populations of problem*

> *drinkers, tends to regard alcohol*
> *use as wholly inadvisable.*
>
> *The other trend is based on both a*
> *realistic acknowledgment of drink-*
> *ing as a deeply ingrained social*
> *practice within Western cultures*
> *and a willingness to consider the*
> *evidence that moderate drinking*
> *may be beneficial. The present*
> *study offers further support for the*
> *latter trend.*

Akers and La Greca (Pittman and White 1991) report the widely recognized reality that " . . . the major findings from past survey research is that the percentage of respondents who report drinking and heavy drinking decreases with age. Surveys of local, regional and national samples have consistently found drinking behavior to be negatively associated with age."

This observation is hardly revolutionary. Older people generally have less discretionary income to spend on drinking. Older folks grow more conservative in all matters.

Withholding information on the benefits of drinking for the elderly makes no sense as this group is the least likely to succumb to addictive drinking. The authors conclude:

*Transition from lifelong abstention
to problem drinking as a means of
coping with the stress of old age is
a very rare phenomenon. If late
onset drinking ever does occur, it is
most likely to occur in those older
adults who enter later life with a
predisposition for heavy drinking.
It is not likely to be provoked by
stressful life events. The elderly
are, by and large, quite capable of
dealing with them without recourse
to alcohol.*

It's been written . . .

The prohibitionists exploited the medical and sexual terrors of the people of America in order to further their cause. In the course of this indoctrination, they were aided by the findings of research and the dicta of doctors. They used every means of propaganda to abolish the saloons.

*Andrew Sinclair, Era of Excess, Harper Colophon
Books, New York 1962*

Chapter 11

Drinking and nutrition

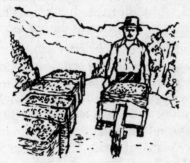

There is no medical evidence of adverse effects of moderate drinking on human nutrition. To the contrarty, there are many anecdotal references to its positive impact (American Heart Association 1986, Ferrence 1985, Forsham 1987, Fraenkel-Conrat 1988, Gastineau 1979, Katz 1986, Sarley 1969, Turner 1977, Turner 1981, Olsen 1985 and Nielsen 1987).

Many papers detail how *excessive drinking* can interfere with vitamin and mineral assimilation. One manifestation of overdrinking is the loss of appetite. Heavy drinking provides more calories than a body needs. An alcoholic who consumes a full bottle of spirits daily ingests more than 4000 calories from that source alone. Since alcohol calories cannot be deposited as fat, they are used to energize the body. They also create a false sense of fullness in the heavy drinker. In contrast, a moderate drinker consuming about 400 alcohol calories daily has plenty of appetite for a balanced diet.

There is some evidence (Turner 1981) that alcohol calories are less efficient as an energy source than other foods. Controlled experiments reveal less weight gain from excess alcohol than in excessive consumption of other forms of food. One researcher (La Porte 1980) estimates that American drinkers get about 8 percent of caloric intake from alcohol.

Whatever the actual amount, it is obvious that alcohol is a supplemental source of non-carbohydrate energy, especially for diabetics (Farsham 1987). It can be an ancillary source of vitamins and trace minerals (Gastineau 1979, Katz 1986 and Nielsen 1987), and ethanol can help to catalyze extra vitamins and minerals. Alcoholic beverages may also provide fat-free, low sodium energy (Turner 1981).

The adverse effects of drinking on nutrition are nearly universally correlated with abusive levels of consumption (Eckhard 1981). Overdrinking interferes with the normal patterns of absorption of vitamins and minerals. Poor eating habits among heavy drinkers exacerbates the already nutrition-poor diet.

By contrast, alcoholic beverages are used in therapy for both the young and the aging who lack appetite (Mishara 1980 and Sarley 1969). By stimulating saliva flow in the mouth and gastric juices in the stomach, alcohol tends to increase true appetite and the desire to eat. Patients administered small amounts of wine or beer in hospitals and nursing homes uniformly demonstrate increased sociability and self esteem, both of which are vital to a healthy appetite and balanced nutrition.

Nutrition and toxicity

Perhaps the most exciting work being done in the nutrition field is that which relates toxicity in alcohol to the diet. This work is being accomplished largely by Veterans' Administration researchers on rats. It indicates that toxic effects of drinking may be controlled by managing levels of intake of carbohydrates. Not surprisingly, this avenue of research is controversial and, as in the case of the French paradox, has gained scant interest or funding from governmental or private research agencies. Apparently the premise that alcohol toxicity and damage

could be alleviated by diet threatens the
current political thinking of neodrys that
alcohol is always *ipso facto* toxic and
damaging. In a recent paper (Sankaran
1992), the authors found:

> *Adverse effects observed in
> alcoholic rats are often attributed
> to alcohol per se. Alcoholic liver
> damage, however, can be avoided
> by modulating nutritional factors
> despite high blood alcohol con-
> centrations.*

The key research premise is that
abnormally high alcohol diets fed animals
reduces the intake of carbohydrates and that
this factor contributes largely to the toxicity.
Consider what these findings could mean to
the alcoholism and fetal syndrome fields.
High food intake could lessen or eliminate
some of the damaging effects.

But we won't ever find out if a pessimistic
attitude prevails in the federal agencies
which control research funding.

Chapter 12

Other positive aspects

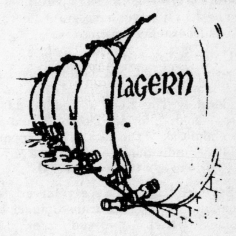

Researchers who observe strong associations between frequent drinking and apparent good health are justifiably cautious about establishing direct causal links between the two (American Heart Association 1987, Bowden 1987, Chalke 1981, Donohue 1986, Emboden 1988, Ferrence 1986, Gusfield 1981 and Longnecker 1988).

Conservatism justified

Despite this understandable caution, there is growing recognition in the medical literature of alcohol as an important element in a healthy lifestyle, a recognition not shared by our federal bureaucracy.

One recent study (Longnecker 1988) reports less hospitalization among both males and females in the population who drink moderately. This study was adjusted for age, race, smoking, former alcoholics and others who might skew the data. These apparently healthier individuals consume, on average, 29 to 42 drinks in a two week period.

Several times I have referred to the Richman and Warren trans-Canada health survey which involved over 17,000 respondents (Richman 1985). The authors found:

> *Moderate to heavy drinkers of liquor and wine (8-34 drinks per week) seem to have had the best morbidity experience with reported morbidity 15-20% below expected levels.*

Any factor that demonstrates better heart health and fewer acute hospitalizations should be of great interest to health conscious America. We are inundated with health fad data. This high correlation of drinking and health can hardly be attributed to chance. At the minimum, it can be said that regular moderate drinking occurs in healthy, well-adjusted people. One must ask why this positive story is de-emphasized or never told by public health spokespeople. Why it never becomes a part of the periodic special reports from NIAAA to Congress.

A long history as medicine

Alcohol is one of the oldest medicines known to man. Through all history, wine and beer were medicines themselves and carriers or menstruums for hundreds of other herbal remedies. Dozens of patent medicines still use alcohol as a base. Medical instruments are cleansed in alcohol solutions. Bacteria cannot survive in alcohol so it is the perfect disinfectant. The human body produces alcohol itself. This is reality not fiction.

Until the discovery of modern wonder drugs, alcohol was the most often-employed drug in the medical pharmacopoeia. It is a travesty that alcoholic beverages were removed from this national directory of useful therapeutic drugs in 1915 under pressure of earlier temperance forces. This catalogue of drugs is maintained by the American Medical Association which, unfortunately, often sides with the anti-drinking lobbies.

There is considerable evidence of a synergistic adaptation of extra vitamins and minerals when alcohol accompanies foods (*Wine and Medical Practice* 1979). In addition to its contributions to cardiovascular health and relief from tension, alcohol has been found to stimulate motility and bile flow, to be a source of energy for diabetics, to enhance kidney function, to increase diuresis, to discourage viral infections as well as to act as an antibiotic.

Two new elements in wine skins have excited great interest. Resveratrol is a phenolic compound produced by the grape vine to fight its diseases. Japanese and Chinese folk medicines employ resveratrol which has been found to lower bad cholesterol. Creasy and Siemann at Cornell University's Department of Fruit and Vegetable Science have isolated resveratrol in a wide range of American red wines as well as in grape juice.

Dr. Terrance Leighton, professor of biochemistry at the University of California, Berkeley, has done pioneer work in isolation of another grape skin compound called quercetin. Digestion enzymes release quercetin from sugar molecules where it becomes a powerful anti-carcinogen. (Leighton 1991)

The social enhancer

Perhaps the greatest contribution to general well-being in moderate alcohol consumption is the least measurable in a purely scientific sense—its enhancement of social communion. An editorial (Chalke 1981) titled "Moderate Drinking—Moderate Damage" in the *British Journal on Alcohol and Alcoholism* describes this holistic dimension of drinking:

> *It is important to acknowledge that drinking by most members of society is not accompanied by problems and may ease the loneliness of old age, the burden of intolerable pain, foster healthy psycho-sexual attitudes or encourage social intercourse.*

A ten year study in Alameda County,
California (Breslow 1980) of seven *good
health practices* found that persons taking
one to two drinks at a time had lesser
mortality rates than those abstaining or those
consuming over four drinks at one time.

A nation of nosophobes

Dr. Elizabeth Whelan of the American
Council on Science and Health describes the
fear of drinking as "nosophobia"—the fear of
what *might* happen—an anxiety that can be
debilitating (Whelan 1984):

> *Nosophobics are everywhere. They
> dominate the airwaves, the
> electronic media. They work for
> self-appointed consumer advocacy
> groups. They have infiltrated high
> level offices of our regulatory
> agencies. If you are having a
> temporary lapse on exactly what
> nosophobia is, let me remind you
> that it is like hypochondria, but it
> is different. Hypochondriacs think
> they are sick. Nosophobics think
> they will in the future be sick, be-
> cause of the lurking factors in the
> environment in which they live.
> Nosophobics have been in ecstasy*

> *in the past decade or so—there is so*
> *much to worry about, so many vil-*
> *lains out there ready to get us, so*
> *much bad news about the state of*
> *health in America.*

A leading authority on addiction observes that millions among us drink regularly without the slightest danger of addiction (Peele 1987) ". . . 25 billion individual occasions in a year when Americans drink alcohol, only a minute percentage—even among those designated as problem drinkers—lead to uncontrolled behavior."

The best advice is to relax, to remain moderate in all things and to enjoy life. In *Health Fact, Health Fiction, Getting Through the Media Maze,* Dr. Robert Taylor (Taylor 1990) advises not to worry:

> *It's important to learn how to*
> *evaluate medical evidence . . . Your*
> *health is far too important to pay*
> *attention to everything you are told*
> *. . . To pursue certain health*
> *practices or to spend a lot of effort*
> *avoiding certain risks is, at best, a*
> *waste of time and, at worst, a*
> *health hazard in its own right.*

It's been written . . .

When alcohol is judged, little regard is paid to its beneficial effects when it is taken in socially acceptable doses. It is not even condemned because of its side effects, which are minimal in small doses, but only because of its toxicity when taken in overdosage; no other pharmacological active substance is judged in this way and there are very few if any entries in the British Pharmacopoeia which would escape castigation if they were. Even water when taken in gross overdosage can, and a few times each year does, kill.

Thomas Stuttaford, M.D., in Drinking to Your Health, Social Affairs Unit, London 1989

Part IV

The

Bad

News

Chapter 13

Alcoholism and alcohol abuse

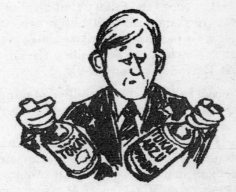

Government statistics on drinking are often exaggerated and overdrawn. Nothing ever gets better according to Health and Human Services. Despite millions of dollars spent on research and prevention, we are told the numbers of abusers are on the increase. Everything's bad.

HHS estimates that there are up to 18 million adults (18 years and above) who have drinking problems (Bowen 1987). The

department also claims that as many as 4.6
million or 3 out of 10 adolescents have serious
health problems from drinking. Drinking is
blamed and not single-parenting,
homelessness, indifferent schooling and drug
infested neighborhoods. Drink's the problem.

HHS echoes the fallacy that alcohol abuse
costs are as much as $130 billion even though
their own paid consultant recently reported
true costs closer to $50 billion (Heien 1989,
Katz 1987, Josephson 1980).

A cost to society of fifty billion is significant
enough. Whatever the true costs of
abuse—and no one disputes their reality or
their enormity—the government is
overstating them. HHS agencies never define
"problem drinking" or "health problems" in
precise scientific terms. As long as HHS
maintains the lie that two drinks a day is
"heavy drinking" and that all drinking is "risk
taking," they can calculate all manner of
fictions.

According to carefully documented
research (Rorabaugh 1979), the per capita
consumption of alcohol since 1860 has
remained within a very narrow range.
Though there are changes—particularly as
the numbers of young adults rise and fall—
total abuse today is close to that of one

hundred years ago. Overdrinking, then, is *endemic* and is closely related to population shifts. The Gallup company reported in 1939 that 58% of Americans claimed to be drinkers. In 1990, Gallup found 57% to be drinkers.

The profile of an average drinker is known. Typical drinkers are men, under the age of 50, Catholics, those living on either coast, and those with higher levels of education and higher incomes. Non-drinkers more often are women, older Americans, Protestants, less well-educated, those having lower incomes and those who live in the Midwest and South.

The barrage of negative propaganda about drinking by HHS is having an effect on public opinion. One question asked each year by Gallup's pollsters is: "Has drinking been a cause of trouble in your family?" From the 1950s to the 1970s, the number who answered yes was under 20%. Since 1985 the "yes" responses have risen as high as 24%. The Just Say No propaganda has worked.

Use and abuse

Since the federal government is the primary source of information on alcohol use and abuse, the media, Congress and the public will, in all likelihood, continue to misperceive these issues until HHS begins to distinguish between use and abuse.

"The Beneficial Side of Moderate Alcohol Use" (Turner 1981) makes this vital distinction:

> *This paper and a previous one by*
> *the senior author and his*
> *associates emphasize that the*
> *long-term effects of alcohol depend*
> *largely on the usual quantity of*
> *intake. In general, chronic ill-*
> *effects are restricted to heavy*
> *drinking, 80 g daily [80 grams at*
> *an average of 14 grams of absolute*
> *alcohol per drink equals 5.7 drinks*
> *daily or more.]*

Classic alcoholism, as defined by the American Medical Association (AMA), is a disease with specific behavioral dimensions and symptoms (*Manual on Alcoholism* 1968). Here is the AMA's definition:

> *Alcoholism is an illness charac-*
> *terized by preoccupation with*
> *alcohol and loss of control over its*
> *consumption such as to lead*
> *usually to intoxication if drinking*
> *is begun; by chronicity; by*

> *progression; and by tendency*
> *toward relapse.*
> *It is typically associated with*
> *physical disability and impaired*
> *emotional, occupational, and/or*
> *social adjustments as a direct*
> *consequence of persistent and*
> *excessive use of alcohol.*

The AMA pamphlet recognizes that any definition of alcoholism will be controversial because the behavior pattern is so complex. But the AMA stresses the characteristic inability of alcoholics to control their actions—thereby distinguishing between those with the addictive "disease" and those who willfully abuse.

The disease concept of alcoholism is controversial (Fingarette 1988). A primary criticism is its assertion that individuals cannot control their behavior. Yet, if alcoholism is a disease, it is one without a pathogen or virus. One author explains this controversial concept as follows (Vogler 1982):

> *Most alcohol counselors support the*
> *disease approach, yet unlike other*
> *diseases, alcoholism cannot be*
> *"caught" through biological means;*

> *there is no alcoholism virus, fungus
> or germ. . . . It is not carried by
> parasites. . . . you cannot sneeze
> and give someone alcoholism . . .
> You cannot get alcoholism
> accidentally. . . . and you are not
> born with it as some would claim.*

To further complicate the discussion, a substantial body of research now seeks to define a biological explanation for alcoholism. The current director of NIAAA, Enoch Gordis, correctly stresses the need for more research on both genetic predisposition and environmental influences (Gordis 1987). But, as yet, biology alone cannot be held accountable for overdrinking. The genetic (*Alcoholism Report,* 1987) findings are confounded by the fact that many who have these isolated genetic markers do not become alcoholic and many others with no genetic pre-disposition succumb to the disease.

Environment a predictor

It is likely that an interplay of heredity and environmental factors trigger latent abuse tendencies in some individuals. Some studies have identified chemistry patterns in brain cells of offspring of alcoholics and marker genes which influence synapses. Still,

environment remains the important
predictor of alcoholism (Harburg 1982):

> *. . . whereas most offspring of*
> *moderate drinkers drink moderate-*
> *ly, most children of heaviest*
> *drinkers also drink moderately and*
> *there are more abstainers' offspring*
> *who drink than who abstain. . . .*
> *even alcoholic parental drinking*
> *only weakly invites imitation by off-*
> *spring.*

The disease concept of alcoholism suffers
because it is simplistic and because it ignores
the role of personal responsibility. If alcohol
is to *blame,* then *alcohol* is also the *cause* in
accidents, robberies, suicides, wife-beatings
and all sorts of social mayhem.

That's what HHS and NIAAA imply in
their series of reports to Congress on alcohol
and health and in other official publications.
They *blame* alcohol for morbidity, death, lost
employment, crime, fires and so on rather
than the perpetrators. This may give comfort
to the neodry cause, but it is scientific
sophistry—a deception in which,
unfortunately, the media warmly cooperates.

Alcohol doesn't jump from the bottle into the mouth and cars don't steer themselves into ditches. People must be made responsible for overdrinking and their ensuing loss of productivity, suicides and accidents. The individual is the cause not the drink.

Fingarette holds the disease concept to be pure myth. He points to its lack of acceptance in the research community (Fingarette 1988):

> *And yet, no leading research authorities accept the classic disease concept. . . . The pattern of chronic heavy drinking seems at least somewhat analagous to these other patterns of behavior, all of which we tend to refer to as addictions, compulsions, or dependence.*

Some feel that our era should be tabbed the *addiction era.* Personal responsibility for aggressive acts are shifted more and more to outside forces. Peele (Peele 1987) contends :

> *I believe that addiction is the central theme our culture uses to explain and attack drug use of which it disapproves, and that the promotion of addictive imagery has*

> *major consequences for amount,*
> *style and results of drug use.*

As these critics point out, drys blame
alcohol (the agent) instead of overdrinking
(by the host). In the most comprehensive and
lengthy study of alcoholism ever conducted,
researchers traced a sample group for over
forty years. Vaillant provides important
insights from this study in *The Natural
History of Alcoholism.* The author points to
ethnic and behavioral patterns as the most
important influences (Vaillant 1983):

> *First, future alcoholics are more
> likely to come from ethnic groups
> that tolerate adult drunkenness but
> that discourage children and
> adolescents from learning safe
> drinking practices (such as
> consumption of low-proof alcoholic
> beverages at ceremonies and with
> meals). Thus parents and
> grandparents of the alcoholics in
> our samples were more likely to
> have been born in English-speaking
> countries than in Mediterranean
> countries.*

When was the last time you heard a government official supporting the training of youth in responsible drinking. Not likely! HHS adamantly pursues its "no use" policy for the young. According to the findings of Vaillant's 40-year study, the control of availability agenda proposed by government today, the raising of the minimum drinking age and the defamation of all alcohol usage is likely to have one *adverse* impact on drinking patterns. It's likely to increase abusive behavior, particularly in the young.

Drinking patterns

The AMA alcoholism pamphlet observes there are four common reasons for drinking, all of which may be acceptable in appropriate circumstances.

First, there is drinking as *religious exercise*. Next there is *ceremonial* drinking such as the toasting at diplomatic events and weddings. Then there is the drinking which most of us do called *utilitarian* drinking—that which accompanies eating and social events. The cocktail party is the quintessential utilitarian drinking event.

Finally, there is *hedonistic* drinking or that done purely for the intellectual and physical enjoyment of the beverage itself. A wine tasting party or a festive meal may involve several or all of these categories. None of these drinking exercises are intrinsically evil, but each one can be carried to excess.

The danger of our national drinking ambivalence is highlighted in a paper titled "Alcohol and Alcoholism" published by the National Institute of Mental Health (NIMH). It states:

> *... the rate of alcoholism is low in those groups in which the drinking customs, values and sanctions are well-established, known to and agreed upon by all, and consistent with the rest of the culture. By contrast, the rate tends to be high in groups with marked ambivalence toward alcohol—with no agreed upon ground rules.*

Abuse on downtrend

It may come as a shock, but even HHS publications admit that problem drinking among adults is trending down. Abusive drinking is expected to drop from the current estimated 10 percent of the drinking population (a questionable estimate to begin with) to 8 percent through the 1990s.

Studies by the National Highway Traffic Safety Administration (Katz 1987) report that the number of fatally injured intoxicated drivers has dropped more than ten percent as has the number of fatalities among youthful drivers.

Similarly, adolescent abuse is expected soon to drop to levels comparable to the mid-1970s. HHS surveys today reveal that 69 percent of youth abstain from drinking altogether; 89 percent abstain from marijuana; and 99 perccnt from heroin.

There is no distinction in government reports between parent-supervised and illegal youthful drinking. Many among the 31 percent of adolescents who report drinking on surveys are doing so in parentally supervised situations. These are truly life-training exercises. Training the young in responsible consumption. It is a scandal that HHS does not separate this use from illegal use.

The *Just Say No* literature distributed in schools encourages children of all ages to pressure their parents not to smoke or to drink, making no essential distinction between those two substances or between a beer and cocaine.

This government pressure (yes, public schools are part of government) discourages parents from passing on their own moderate drinking habits and patterns. The "alcohol and other drugs" campaign fails to recognize the responsible drinking pattern of the majority of adults in society. Anderson suggests the consequences of this policy (Anderson 1989) of less is better:

> *There is considerable disagreement*
> *among the experts about limits . . .*
> *but what is immediately striking is*
> *their extremism. They are extreme*
> *in that they have moved well across*
> *the range of consumption and are*
> *getting close to zero. . . . If they*
> *continue in their current direction*
> *at their recent pace, they will be*
> *tantamount to teetotalism in a*
> *couple of decades . . . the ladies*
> *have only one small glass to go.*

Abuse categories

We already know a lot about which groups in society are more likely to abuse alcohol. As the average age in America rises, there is less alcohol abuse because there are fewer upper-teens and young adults who do most of the public abusing.

Alcoholism and abuse have a high correlation with the socially disadvantaged, high risk, inner-city groups (Harburg 1982). The disadvantaged, the criminal, and those who live apart from the mainstream of society are consistent abusers (*Inner City Youth* 1988).

HHS reports alcohol abuse as high as 55 percent among the economically disadvantaged; 42 percent among children of substance abusers; 29 percent among juvenile delinquents; and 39 percent among drug users. No surprises here.

Abuse is not alcoholism

While millions in the world go to bed hungry, our teenage population is estimated to have a $40 billion annual disposal income. The mirror image of deprivation in our society is affluence. Poor black kids in the cities and rich white kids in the suburbs both are at greater risk of abusing alcohol and illicit drugs.

Aside from these "high risk" populations, the broad range of social drinkers are not potential addicts. Abusers are not necessarily addicts either. They can quit abusing when they put their minds to the task. Over 50 million people in the U.S. have quit smoking.

Thousands of servicemen used cocaine freely while in Viet Nam but voluntarily stopped the use upon return to the states.

Alcohol abusers can, and often do, stop their abusive patterns for extended periods. Frequently public intoxication and anti-social behavior are often manifestations of transitory personal stress. Abusive drinking is any consumption which is socially offensive or dangerous to self or others. Abusive drinking fails to meet the AMA's definition of classic alcoholism.

Abuse may be periodic or chronic but the causes of the abuse often lie in deep-rooted psychological problems and not in the bottle itself. Anthropologists report more of this kind of public abuse in societies where norms of drinking are uncertain (Heath 1987):

> *When alcohol-related problems do occur, they are clearly linked with modalities of drinking, and usually also with values, attitudes, and norms about drinking.*

The legal drinking age of twenty-one and the *macho* image of "holding one's liquor contribute to abuse (*Wine and Medical Practice* 1979).

Classic alcoholism, as defined by the AMA, affects a relatively small segment of the drinking population—something in the range of 5 percent. Abusive or problem drinking may well involve another fluctuating 5 percent of that population. These percentages have changed very little in this long century of drinking ambivalence. HHS reports a "growing alcohol problem" (Bowen 1987), but the NIAAA's own in-house epidemiologists predict no substantial change in abuse patterns until the 18 year-old population again rises around 1995 (*Demographic Trends* 1987). Obviously, there is a great deal of bureaucratic puffery in abuse data.

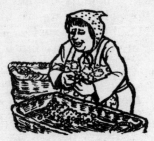

Women at particular risk

There is new interest in female abusive drinking. The liberation of women has brought new drinking problems. About 5 percent (Lex 1988) of women are found now

to be alcohol dependent. Paternal alcoholism
may be a more important criterion for women
than for men. A study of cognitive
performance holds (Lex 1988)

> *In a national survey sample, more*
> *women than men reported having*
> *alcoholic fathers . . . and*
> *prevalence of alcoholism in fathers*
> *of female alcoholics in treatment*
> *is as high as 61%.*

Another study revealed a slower rate of
oxidation of ethanol in women (Fredda 1990)
because of lower concentrations of water and
a slower enzymatic response to ethanol. A
range of studies finds women to be more
susceptible to alcoholism, to high blood
pressure related to drinking, and to liver
cirrhosis. These factors suggest lower levels
of consumption among female consumers.

NIAAA admits benefits

A recent NIAAA monograph "Alcohol
Alert" (Gordis 1992)provides a grudging
recognition of some benefits to be derived
from drinking responsibly (Gordis 1992).
Director Enoch Gordis states:

> *A review of the literature suggests
> that lower levels of alcohol
> consumption can reduce stress;
> promote conviviality and pleasant
> and carefree feelings; and
> decreased tension, anxiety, and self-
> consciousness."*

The paper concludes that young adults can be told that "moderate drinking would probably not be harmful." While the Gordis paper represents a long overdue recognition of the obvious, I wonder when NIAAA will loosen its purse strings and spend some research dollars defining those benefits.

Finally, there is no better advice than to never exceed a .55 BAC as found in *The Better Way To Drink.* (Vogler and Bartz 1982):

> *In summary, since a BA above 55
> (BAC above .55) loses its positive
> quality for most drinkers, and a
> rising BA feels much better than a
> falling BA, we can conclude that
> the most satisfying and successful
> way to drink is to start completely
> sober, drink for 30-45 minutes, and
> back down. That's the ideal way.*

Chapter 14

Drinking and liver disease

Ethanol enters the bloodstream and travels to the liver where it is metabolized into acetaldehyde, then to acetate, and finally to carbon dioxide and water which is expelled.

This metabolism occurs at the rate of about 10 grams an hour. Because the liver is the main organ for metabolizing alcohol, it is particularly vulnerable to alcohol injury or to its toxicity. In large quantities, both ethanol and acetaldehyde may be harmful to the liver, although even among alcohol abusers, liver damage is seldom predictable.

Temperance forces have always used the incidence of liver disease as a barometer of the rate of alcoholism. NIAAA's February 1992 Epidemiology Report indicates a 9.1 per 100,000 death rate from liver cirrhosis, the lowest since 1951. This figure capped a nine year decline. If cirrhosis is the measure, there must fewer alcoholics out there today than ten years ago.

The first sign of alcohol-related liver damage is the accumulation of fat within liver cells, a condition known as fatty liver. In its early stages, fatty liver is reversible through abstinence and it leaves no permanent damage. When the fatty liver condition persists, liver function may diminish and the stage is set for the next level of damage—alcoholic hepatitis. This is characterized by liver inflammation, changes in liver cell structure, and death of liver tissue.

Cirrhosis occurs when scar tissue replaces the dead tissue, disrupting the organ's function and structure. Cirrhosis is the one form of liver damage most directly tied in the public mind to excessive drinking. Cirrhosis is the ninth largest cause of death in the United States (Moore 1987). However, liver cirrhosis occurs in many individuals who do not drink and is avoided by many heavy drinkers so that it is an unreliable measurement for overdrinking (*Wine and Medical Practice* 1979).

Some individuals who consume up to 160 grams of alcohol daily do not become cirrhotic. Malnutrition, common in heavy drinkers, may contribute to the condition. The reasons for this selectivity are unknown. Studies indicate that consumption under the recommended 80 grams per day level presents no danger for cirrhosis but that drinking above that level increases the risk of the disease enormously.

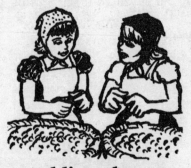

Women and liver damage

Again, there is particular concern about the increased vulnerability in women to liver cirrhosis (Norton 1987) from drinking.

> *The risk of alcohol-related cirrhosis*
> *was significantly increased in*
> *women who consumed 4-6 drinks*
> *(41-60 g of ethanol) daily.*

Others (Selzer 1976) point to differing susceptibilities among nationalities and ethnic groupings. Jews, as example, are rarely cirrhotic regardless of drinking levels. The incidence of cirrhosis has dropped steadily in the United States over the past decade, plummeting over 30 percent to around 10 individuals per 100,000 deaths. Drinking no more than 80 grams per day would further reduce the incidence of liver cirrhosis.

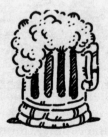

Chapter 15

Drinking and
fetal dysfunctions

The issue of drinking during pregnancy is emotion-laden and clouded by speculative statistics and shrewdly calculated propaganda. Unfortunately, federal and state governments, many state medical societies, and anti-alcohol advocacies have shed more heat than light with their stance for total abstinence during pregnancy.

The fear campaign is misguided. A recent Angus Reid Group survey revealed that 92

percent of the population is aware of fetal
alcohol syndrome. The shame is that most of
what is known is propagandistic and
misleading.

Should pregnant women drink?
Researchers honestly differ on danger levels
during gestation. It is obvious that no one
needs to drink during pregnancy. Any woman
with the slightest doubt about the issue
should simply abstain during the nine
months of pregnancy. The reality is, however,
that many, if not most, practicing physicians
allow moderate drinking after the first
trimester.

FAS a rare phenomenon

Prior to the 1970s, alcohol was thought to
be harmless to the fetus. Intensive research
has now developed a set of symptoms that
relate directly to heavy alcohol ingestion.
FAS, consists of retarded growth, the
development of classic facial anomalies, and
central nervous system dysfunctions. It is
found in a significant number of children of
alcoholic women who drink throughout their
pregnancies (Eckhard 1981).

Classic FAS is rare. As late as 1983,
researchers reported slightly more than 400
cases of FAS worldwide (Rosett 1983):

> *All reported cases of the full FAS*
> *occurred in children of chronic*
> *alcoholic mothers who drank*
> *heavily throughout pregnancy;*
> *none have been reported in children*
> *of women who drank moderately.*

In the *U.S. Journal*, O'Connell found Surgeon General C. Everett Koop's policy of abstinence during pregnancy at odds with a twelve year study on FAS. The NIAAA financed study was conducted at Boston University Medical Center by Rosett and Weiner. He reported their conclusion as (O'Connell 1986):

> *Women place their babies at risk*
> *when they drink five or more*
> *drinks on one occasion. The risks of*
> *drinking three to four drinks in one*
> *sitting are unknown. However,*
> *there is no evidence of damage to*
> *the fetus if a woman chooses to*
> *drink less than one ounce of*
> *absolute alcohol on any given day.*

Rosett and Weiner also found that FAS occurs among only 2 to 10 percent of fully chronic, alcohol-dependent women. Weiner recommends for pregnant women who choose to drink an *upper limit* of one-half of one ounce of absolute alcohol on any single day. This is the equivalent of a single drink. All of the studies concur that FAS is related primarily to very heavy drinking (Plant 1985, Light 1988, Mendelson 1985, and Hamelsmaki 1987) but some (Light 1988) agree with Koop and advise against any drinking:

> *Despite the overwhelming and unequivocal evidence that the drinking of alcohol can and does cause congenital deformities and retardation—even in moderate or small amounts—our cultural imperative that drinking not only is appropriate and even "good" for you, continues to feed an acrimonious debate.*

Fetal alcohol effects

FAS is confused often in the media and in anti-alcohol propaganda with a series of conditions now called fetal alcohol effects (FAE). This condition is apparently much more common (Eckhard 1981, Rosett 1983, Webb 1988 and Graham 1988).

FAE abnormalities are less visually pronounced at birth and include growth retardation, central nervous system involvement and limited facial dysmorphology. FAE may also result from malnutrition, smoking, other drug use and genetics, aside from excessive alcohol during pregnancy.

The incidence of FAE is thought to be more widespread in the United States though this may be a consequence of greater emphasis on the research. One study estimates as many as 36,000 FAE births annually.

Even with FAE, researchers are uncertain as to the specific role of alcohol as a causal factor. One writes "It is important that parents of abnormal children not be burdened with unnecessary guilt for having consumed small amounts of alcohol and not hold themselves responsible for causing anomalies that were actually due to other causes." Also, the attempt to associate any level of drinking as the major source of mental retardation is disputed (Rosett 1983):

> *Many FAS programs have*
> *incorporated this statement in*
> *prevention campaigns. . . . In fact*
> *only 10 percent of the cases of*
> *mental retardation are of known*
> *origin; in 90 percent, the causes*
> *are unknown.*

Many commentators advise a restricted
alcohol intake but do not find specific danger
to the fetus in drinking under two drinks per
day or no more than one ounce of absolute
alcohol (Mills 1987, Rosett 1983 and Webb
1988). One report from a study of 32,870
mothers is typical of these findings (Mills
1987):

> *Total malformation rates were not
> significantly higher among off-
> spring of women who had an
> average of less than one drink per
> day (77.3 / 1000) . . . Likewise,
> major malformations were not in-
> creased in these drinking groups.*

HHS maintains that the risks of
miscarriage or retarded growth rise when a
pregnant woman has as little as one-half to
one ounce of alcohol a week (DHHS and
Eckhard 1981). The HHS publication "My
Baby. . . Strong and Healthy" quotes the
former Surgeon General Koop that, "The
safest choice is not to drink at all during
pregnancy or if you are planning pregnancy."

Continuing studies in dysmorphology
(Graham 1988) report higher incidences of
FAE among mothers who consumed 2 ounces

of absolute alcohol daily (four drinks) prior to the recognition of pregnancy. The pattern of consumption may also make a difference. Regular light drinking may be less harmful on a fetus than the equivalent amount of alcohol consumed in one sitting.

NIAAA and the anti-alcohol lobby use biased, intentionally frightening statistics. According to the public health departments of a dozen states, FAE births are rare. FAS is so rare that most states do not even have specific recording procedures to monitor its incidence.

Figures quoted often in the media are extrapolations from small research studies (Sokol 1980 and Abel 1985). Using a figure of 3,500,000 births, Abel estimates there could be from 1800 to 4000 FAS babies born annually nationwide. Another researcher (Streissguth 1987) enlarges Abel's estimate to 1 in 750 births. This elaboration is boosted once again by NIAAA (*Sixth Special Report to Congress on Alcohol and Health*) "The most common estimate of overall FAS prevalence continues to be 1 to 3 cases per 1,000 live births." *Time* magazine magnifies this into 50,000 babies born with alcohol-related effects.

My own telephone survey of all fifty states revealed a much lower incidence. As example,

Washington State reported 2 FAS babies among over 70,000 births. California, with the best reporting system in the nation, estimates one FAS baby in 10,000 live births.

An important new paper was recently published by two of our nation's prominent FAS researchers (Abel and Sokol 1992) which downsizes both the probable incidence and costs of FAS. "A Revised Conservative Estimate of the Incidence of FAS and its Economic Impact" concludes from prospective studies now completed that the incidence is six times lower than former estimates. The estimated costs dropped from over $300 million to around $75 million.

Rosett and Weiner offer the sagest advice for pregnant women:

> *For the most cautious, abstention
> removes all danger from alcohol . .
> however, the recommendation that
> all women should abstain from
> drinking during pregnancy is not
> based upon scientific evidence . . .
> exaggerating the facts about
> alcohol and pregnancy blurs the
> real dangers of heavy drinking.*

Chapter 16

Drinking, cancer and toxicity

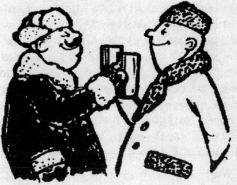

Another neoprohibition scare tactic is the linkage of drinking to cancer.

Committees of the World Health Organization (WHO) are seeking to identify all the elements in modern living which are carcinogenic, mutagenic or toxic. This international exchange of data is coordinated through a committee called the International Agency for Research on Cancer (IARC). This group and some American public health

agencies, such as California's Proposition 65
scientific panel, have placed alcohol on the
lists of potential carcinogens. This is an
arbitrary and capricious misuse of scientific
data. It is but another tool in the campaign to
lower per capita consumption.

Reporting on the California Proposition 65
panel findings, the *San Francisco Chronicle*
(April 23, 1988) said, "Experts Link Booze to
Cancer." *The Los Angeles Times* headline
(April 23, 1988) stated "Alcohol, Cancer
Linked by Governor's Panel." Even though
the undersecretary for Health and Welfare for
California *discounted* the relation of
moderate drinking to cancer, the strong
impression of alcohol as a carcinogen remains
in the public mind.

Breast cancer scare

The scare over breast cancer and drinking
demonstrates how easily the media can
unwittingly distort health dangers and fail to
report subsequent ameliorating research.

In 1987, two articles on breast cancer
appeared in the *New England Journal of
Medicine* (Schatzkin 1987 and Willett 1987).
These and other corroborating studies
(Graham 1987 and Harburg 1982) were
widely reported in the popular media since

they linked even moderate drinking with a higher risk of this form of cancer. "Viewed collectively, they suggest that alcohol intake may contribute to the risk of breast cancer."

The error lies in confusing *association* with *causality*. Alcohol may be a contributing factor, such as in the linkage of alcohol with tobacco induced cancers. Many breast cancer studies find a stronger relationship with dietary fats than with drinking. Subsequent research (Schatzkin 1989a and 1989b) disparaged this relationship:

> *Alcohol consumption was not
> associated with an increased risk of
> breast cancer in this cohort.. . . .
> These findings do not support the
> positive alcohol-breast cancer
> correlation that has been suggested
> in epidemiological studies.*

The one-in-ten cancer statistic

Another widely quoted statistic avers that breast cancer affects one in ten women. Seldom is it reported that epidemiological studies find the one in ten risk occurring in females who survive into their 80s and not in the general population.

Commentary in the professional journals raises questions about the validity of the linkage and the methodology of the two studies. An Australian study reported it to be "at most, qualified" (Rohan 1988), and a study of 1467 women (Harris 1988) found:

> *While these results do not entirely
> rule out a weak association between
> breast cancer and alcohol in
> certain subgroups, neither do they
> provide compelling evidence that
> alcohol has a role in the genesis of
> this malignancy.*

Other researchers have cast doubt on the alcohol/breast cancer link (Harvey 1987, Herbert 1987, Pollack 1984 and Webster 1983). An exchange of correspondence in the *New England Journal of Medicine* (1987) referred to a ten year study in Sweden which was unable to confirm the link. Other American studies which suggest stress and psychosocial factors as covariant factors are not often cited.

Given the inevitable sensationalism in media coverage, it is important that the NIAAA and other public health agencies maintain an objective stance in their publications about breast cancer, and all other cancers that relate in any way to drinking.

Heavy drinking and cancer

Apart from breast cancer, there is no doubt that heavy alcohol consumption (Eckhard 1981)—often combined with smoking—has been causally correlated with cancers of the mouth, larynx, pharynx, esophagus, lung, bladder, colon, rectum, and liver. The author concludes:

> *The means by which alcohol might*
> *exert a carcinogenic effect in man*
> *are unknown.*

There is intense interest now in exploring a possible role of drinking and colonic polyps as possible cancer precursors. One study (Cope 1991) found the risk of polyps increased at every level of drinking. Another (Choi 1991) found increased risk of cancer of the esophagus, rectum and liver in men who consumed more than two drinks a day. In most of these studies, cancer is associated with heavy drinking, smoking, and malnutrition. The evidence implicating lower levels of alcohol consumption has been inconsistent.

Alcohol to date has not been found to be a direct carcinogen though recent studies suggest such a link (Fraenkel-Conrat 1988 and Herbert 1987) through the action of acetaldehyde on human DNA. Substances in alcoholic beverages called congeners may be carcinogenic. Heavy drinkers are often heavy smokers, and the alcohol and tobacco may act synergistically to boost cancer risk. Whatever the reason, the risk of cancer to certain organs does seem to increase as alcohol consumption increases, although the threshold at which that risk rises meaningfully has not been determined. Cancer incidence is lower in abstemious populations in this country, such as Seventh Day Adventists, but this group usually avoids tobacco as well.

World Health Organization bias

There is no valid link between alcohol and cancer despite the determinations of the California Proposition 65 and the IARC scientific panels. Nearly the entire range of foods in our diet contain some potential carcinogens (Whelan 1989 and Ames 1986). Experts question (Rubin 1988) motivation of the World Health Organization's attempts to associate alcohol and cancer:

> *At least two types of bias may occur
> in epidemiological studies—selec-
> tion bias and reporting bias. Both
> seriously complicate the reliability
> of the epidemiological studies
> reviewed by IARC.*

Urethane controversy overblown

Another controversy involves the natural
production of urethane in selected types of
fermented and distilled beverages. Urethane
has induced cancer in laboratory animals in
mega-doses. The Food and Drug
Administration has reached agreements with
the distilled spirits and wine industries on
acceptable parts-per-million levels.

Ironically, the Center for Science in the
Public Interest and other anti-alcohol forces
have pressed this case against the beverage
industry while ignoring the presence of
urethane in other fermented foods such as
bread, yogurt, pickles and sauerkraut.

Foods undergo adaptation

It is important for the public to gain a
broader perspective on the reports on
cancer-causing agents in the beverages and
foods which we routinely consume.

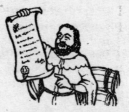

Carcinogens abound in nature. Many of the minerals and salts we depend on for health (Ames 1987) are carcinogenic such as lead, cadmium, beryllium, nickel and chromium. More than 5,000 chemicals found in the common foods we eat could be carcinogenic if taken at the excessive levels fed to laboratory animals.

In the last several hundred years, we have added a number of new toxic plants to our cuisines. Each requires a period of human adaptation. Among these are coffee, potatoes, jalapenas, tomatoes and kiwi. The human system slowly adapts to accommodate new mutagens and carcinogens from edibles. The American Council on Science and Health has published a Thanksgiving Day menu listing the carcinogens in our regular diet. Carcinogenic foods include celery, parsley, spinach, figs, cocoa powder, cola, peanut butter, bread, cheese and fruit. Potatoes are also highly toxic. Alfalfa sprouts could cause lupus, and our barbecue charcoal is one-hundred percent carcinogenic.

Professor Bruce Ames, noted cancer expert at the University of California, sums up this overweening fear of cancer and other pollutants this way:

> *I guess people can say, "If there's any risk, I'll chuck it." But there's no life at all without some risk. Every organism pollutes. You breathe carcinogens out of your mouth after you drink a beer. Sunshine is a carcinogen, but do you want to put up an umbrella every time you cross the street? Then you run the risk of poking someone's eye out.*

An Ames "risk chart" rates the cancer hazard among foods. It places alcohol relatively high but qualifies that risk if used in moderate dosages.

> *The possible hazard of alcohol is enormous relative to that from the intake of synthetic chemical residues. If alcohol, trichloroethylene, DDT, and other presumptive nongenotoxic*

> *carcinogens are active at high doses*
> *because they are tumor promoters,*
> *the risk from low doses may be*
> *minimal.*

What is needed among the public is a strong dose of good old common sense in evaluating data on drinking and cancer. Without question, heavy drinking and its attendant consumptive lifestyle, particularly smoking and poor nutrition, can increase the risk of various cancers. To this point, no one has discovered a definitive link between moderate drinking and cancer. These complex and often speculative findings contain great uncertainties and irresolution.

The linkages can become silly and superfluous. One project found that barmaids had higher mortality from cirrhosis but lower proportional death from breast cancer. Another, (*New England Journal of Medicine* 1987) even suggested that the presence of sulfites in wines, a chemical which now must be reported as hazardous on labels, may help to prevent cancer.

> *These studies suggested the*
> *hypothesis that the relatively high*
> *sulfite content of wine as compared*
> *with other alcoholic beverages*

might have a protective or mitigating role with respect to carcinogens.

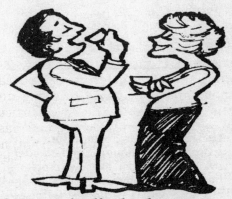

Moderates in little danger

Common sense suggests that moderate drinkers are in no great danger from drinking. HHS should reassure the public against undue alarm. Its silence on this important issue is one more evidence of the anti-drinking bent within our federal bureaucracy. An anonymous wag put these incessant alcohol and food scares into humorous perspective:

> *Only Irish Coffee provides in a single glass all four essential food groups: alcohol, caffeine, sugar and fat.*

It's been written

Utilizing friends', supporters', and patrons' assertions as independent evidence to support their own programs has been a common practice in the alcohol programs of the past 100 years. The process takes on rather frightening overtones when government agencies control not only their own action policies but also the so-called independent research.

Selden D. Bacon, "An Old Warrior Looks at the New" in **Alcohol: The Development of Sociological Perspectives on Use and Abuse**, P. Roman, Ed., Rutgers Center of Alcohol Studies, New Brunswick 1991

Chapter 17

Drinking and driving

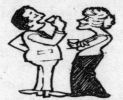

The statistics generated by the federal government on drinking and driving are overladen with questionable assumptions. The tragedy is that Congress, state legislatures and police departments all feed out of the same trough. No one questions the assumptions or clarifies their meanings.

Americans hear and read that about fifty percent of the deaths on our highways are "alcohol-related." Alcohol-related can mean as little as an officer smelling alcohol on the breath of any occupant of an automobile.

Recent research published by Ottawa's Traffic Injury Research Foundation (Simpson and Mayhew 1992) focuses on the real predator in this mix. The study found "hard core drinkers" to be the most productive target of legislation and control. While 46 percent of fatally injured drivers had been drinking, "the overwhelming majority of fatally injured drivers—about 80% of them—had BACs in excess of the legal limit. ... 64% had alcohol levels of .15 or above and 40% had BACs over .20." Forty percent had blood alcohol levels double legal intoxication!

While alcohol-involved deaths are numerous and tragic, the *reality* is far from the *perception*. Approximately 31% of our fatal automobile accidents involve drunken drivers and one-third of the injuries are related to alcohol abuse (Colquitt 1987 and Pisani 1987). That's a lot but it's not 50 percent. In 1985, more than 14,500 drunken drivers were involved in fatal car crashes, and more than 18,000 deaths occur each year from alcohol-associated traffic accidents (Gundby 1987).

Aside from the fatalities, over 3 million people suffer injuries each year and a staggering $74.2 billion drain occurs each year to our economy in crash costs (Turner 1977). Aside from the drinking issue, the pain, misery, and financial drain from universal automobile use are phenomenal. Yet, isn't it strange that we accept the costs and carnage in exchange for the privilege and independence of personal transportation. It's a given in our society that the benefits of the car outweigh the very real costs.

No one excuses or condones driving when impaired from alcohol or any other substance. But in recent years scant public attention is focused on the other two-thirds—the "sober" fatalities. We have the *fewest* highway deaths per million miles traveled of any nation in the world. We cannot reduce accidents to zero. We are doing a good job.

Traffic deaths through the first six months of 1991 were the lowest in years according to an article in the *Journal of the American Medical Association* (AMA 1992). National Highway Traffic Safety Administration (NHTSA) figures reveal a nearly ten-percent drop from 44,529 to 41,150.

One telling commentary in the article cited 2,734,000 road fatalities since Henry Bliss became the first in New York City on September 13, 1899. We have killed and maimed each other relentlessly ever since the car was introduced to society.

NHTSA has set a worthy goal of 26,000 deaths by the year 2000. While we strive as a nation to reach that objective, we must keep in mind that as long as people, alcohol, and a range of legal and illegal drugs are in common usage, fatalities will inevitably occur. It serves no public purpose to presume that we can *eliminate* drunken driving any more than we can eliminate *careless* driving.

Drunken driving profile known

Traffic accidents and other violent forms of trauma are among the worst health hazards associated with alcohol abuse. Drunken driving is a difficult problem to solve because the people arrested for it cover a large social spectrum. DWI convictions come from all walks of life and all social strata. We have an established offender profile for the drunken drivers. We do know that certain sub-populations are causing *most* of the problems (Youngers 1990):

> *The fatal drunk driver is most
> likely in the range of 18 to 34 years
> of age and male. The chances are 4
> out of 5 that he is unmarried. He is
> apt also to be an unskilled or semi-
> skilled laborer. He probably had a
> previous DWI conviction, a prior
> accident, a prior moving violation,
> and a prior revoked or suspended
> license.*

Rehabilitation programs for DWI offenders have been uniformly disappointing. There remains a very high rate of recidivism. In one study, 50 percent of high-risk drivers had severe alcohol problems and most were driving with revoked licenses (Scales 1984). There is no mechanism in society to date, public or private, to harness this large and disparate population of repeat offenders. And throwing them in jail doesn't work as the Scandanavians have discovered. You soon run out of jails.

In "DWI—Are We Off Track" Klein points to the futility of laws downsizing the BAC levels as passed in Oregon and California (Klein 1992). "Drunk driving is symptomatic of the larger problem of chronic alcoholism. Greater benefits could be realized by focusing new resources on programs involving prevention."

Simpson and Mayhew (1992) advise a new focus on the hard-core drinker:

> *Technological approaches to keep suspended offenders from driving may need to be part of an overall strategy to reduce impaired driving.*

These researchers found that "For example, high-BAC drivers are more likely to be aged 25 to 34, to have a history of previous DWI convictions as well as license suspensions, to have been driving without a valid license and to be involved in single-vehicle collisions." The reality is that a small segment of drivers are causing most of the problem. Government should focus prevention on this group rather than sponsoring feckless campaigns to eliminate any drinking and driving or to reduce the BACs to such a level as to discourage any drinking.

Alcohol the prime scapegoat

Additionally many motorists, young drivers in particular, are poly-drug users (Williams 1984). Over 20 different drugs were found in the bodies of young, male highway victims in an 18 month California study of highway deaths. Two or more drugs were found in 43 percent of these 440 bodies. In many accidents, alcohol is blamed exclusively since it is the only drug for which there is an available field test. Alcohol impairment is the major—but not the only—cause of injury and death on our roadways. While California may not be typical, the study illustrates a problem.

One road test conducted by British patrol officers found that the common flu bug impaired drivers to the approximate level of .08 BAC. The real problem is *impaired* driving with emphasis on drunken-driving.

Progress unrecognized

Very substantial progress has been achieved over the past two decades in highway safety. Intensive safety education in the United States has brought about the lowest annual death rate per hundred million miles traveled of any country on earth. That's the truth. It is safer to drive here than anywhere else. Dr. Simpson points to these as the *easy* gains. The difficult work lies ahead.

Yet alcohol-involved accidents and deaths have dropped along with the overall improvement in highway safety. The number of drunken drivers involved in fatal crashes declined by more than 2,000 between 1982 and 1985. This reduction can be attributed to many factors including increased public awareness, and more severe sentences handed down to those convicted. Other elements in this success story are reduced speed limits, safer cars, better road lighting and community-wide systems approaches to safety (Ross 1984). Ironically, Congress recently *increased* highway speed limits in the face of overwhelming evidence that new rates of death will occur. It is conservatively estimated that hundreds of deaths are occurring each year from these higher speeds.

Drunks kill drunks

The publicity surrounding drinking and driving misleads in one respect. It fails to define clearly the victim population. The majority of deaths are the drunks or those— like the recently killed baseball manager Billy Martin—who ride with drunks.

One Department of Transportation study reported that 52 percent of deaths in 1983 were drunk drivers, another 20 percent were willing passengers of drunk drivers, and a final 11 percent were drunk pedestrians. Of the 25,000 alcohol-related deaths that year, only 2,550 (O'Neill 1987) were truly innocent victims such as those represented by MADD.

Some researchers suggest novel approaches to deterrence (Asch 1985) such as delaying driver licensing until young people have mastered drinking skills. Others (Ross 1984 and Wagenaar 1983) caution that the universal age of 21 for drinking and more restrictive laws will prove illusory in reducing drunk driving among the teen population.

One comprehensive survey (Sherman 1986) of drunk driving fatalities highlights the inconsistencies and failures of the Department of Transportation's Fatal Accident Reporting System (FARS) upon which the public statistics depend. This report stated that at least 40 states failed to comply with reporting standards. "The FARS data is only as good as what the states supply. With 'garbage' data from the states on alcohol tests, only 'garbage' national estimates of drunk driving can result."

The whole alcohol-related reporting system can be misleading. The National Highway Traffic Safety Administration defines an accident alcohol-related ". . . if a driver or a non-occupant (such as a pedestrian) had a measurable or estimated blood alcohol concentration of .01 percent or above. . ." The reality is that nearly everyone who drinks also drives. The current objective "If you drink, don't drive" is impractical. We used to say "Know your limits." and "Don't drive drunk." These themes make much more sense to a drinking/driving public..

The point is that moderates must question government reporting that systematically overstates drinking's role. Is it done to achieve prohibitionary rather than safety objectives? There's plenty of blame for alcohol to go around. According to Youngers (1991), "A sober driver could hit and kill a drunk driver waiting for a red light to change and the accident will be 'alcohol-related'."

The focus is fuzzy

Even sources as reliable as the American
Council on Science and Health (ACSH 1991)
can become overcautious. Their otherwise
meritorious booklet *The Responsible Use of
Alcohol* is weakened, in my judgment, by an
overdrawn warning. "ACSH recommends
that operators abstain from moderate alcohol
consumption 4-5 hours prior to operating a
vehicle." Very few of us will, so the warning is
specious.

Drunken driving must remain a high
priority focus. But, so must errant driving by
sober people. Highway safety experts (Ross
1984) strongly support deterrence for the
short run but just as strongly advocate new
approaches to safety:

> *Since the practicality of deterrence
> in the long run is questionable and
> its justice arguable, other ap-
> proaches to reduction of death and
> injury. . . ought to be considered by
> policymakers.*

Chapter 18

Other
adverse effects

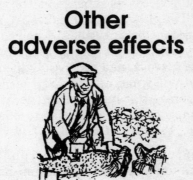

I try never to downplay the terrible ravages of overdrinking. Since many researchers dispute the benefits of drinking, I think their opinions should also be heard (Eckhard 1981, Ferrence 1986 and Knupfer 1987). Knupfer forcefully questions all the benefits reported in the literature from daily drinking:

There is a mistaken notion that some research supports the idea that taking a drink or two every day is good for health. . . It is concluded that the main health and mortality differences, when they do show up, are between drinkers and non-drinkers.

Another commentator (Ferrence 1986) cautions that:

> *. . . on the strength of the available
> evidence, it would be unwise to
> alter either the scientific or public
> policy that might make drinking
> more socially acceptable and
> thereby encourage higher levels of
> consumption.*

Drinking is not for everyone. Even moderates need to be forewarned about the many hazards that their drinking could involve.

The most comprehensive paper I've found concerning the debilitative effects of drinking is "Health Hazards Associated with Alcohol Consumption" (Eckhard 1981) which inventories the physical, social and epidemiological consequences of abusive drinking. The study cites 348 peer-reviewed references. This study begins:

> *Alcohol misuse has a pervasive and
> potentially detrimental effect on the
> body from its point of entry through
> the gastrointestinal tract, to related
> organs such as the liver and
> pancreas.*

The paper concludes with an altogether admirable philosophy:

> *The convivial function of fermented juices has been celebrated in rhyme and song since time immemorial. Alcohol as a food, euphoriant, or social lubricant continues to be an important component of modern society.*

Heavy drinking and nutrition

Heavy drinking and alcoholism have been associated with nutritional deficiencies for several reasons. First, alcoholic beverages tend to be relatively low in nutrients. Second, abusive drinking disrupts the absorption and/or the metabolism of vitamins, minerals, proteins, and carbohydrates, and can damage the digestive tract, leading to nutrient loss through vomiting and diarrhea. Some of the brain damage associated with chronic alcoholism is reversible through abstention and supplements of thiamin (vitamin B-1) but no serious brain damage has been found in moderate drinkers (Bowden 1987).

Heavy drinking has been linked to cardiomyopathy, hypertension (high blood pressure), and an increased risk of stroke. Light to moderate drinking, on the other hand, has been linked to a lowered risk of coronary artery disease, and to fewer heart attacks.

Periodic heavy drinking

True binge drinking has been associated with a condition called "holiday heart syndrome," consisting of heart rhythm disturbances. Much more than the amounts defined herein as moderate must be consumed and over a very short period of time. The syndrome may occur in people who normally drink lightly or moderately, as well as among those who drink heavily. The symptoms are frightening but do not cause lasting damage.

The reports of drinking on the risk of stroke are inconsistent (Donohue 1986). In some studies, stroke risk has increased for people who drink as little as one ounce of absolute alcohol a month, while in others the risk has decreased with an intake of an ounce a day.

Hypertension, or high blood pressure, which raises the risk of stroke, has also been associated with heavy, long-term alcohol consumption. While it is not yet known whether alcohol directly raises blood pressure or if it merely exacerbates hypertension caused by other factors, the evidence to date strongly suggests that heavy consumers run

a greater risk of developing high blood
pressure (Gleiberman 1986). The data are
inconsistent, but risk of chronic hypertension
does not seem to be significant if daily ethanol
intake is less than 40 grams, or three ounces
of 100 proof whiskey (American Heart
Association 1986). Alcohol-induced
hypertension is reversible with abstention.

Too little and too much

The risk of coronary heart disease (CHD)
appears to be lessened by the daily
consumption of one or more ounces of absolute
alcohol. Yet, more than three ounces a day
ushers in the risk of other health problems
that could negate any benefit to the heart.

Prolonged alcoholism can cause serious
damage to the brain and nervous system,
some of which persists even during
subsequent abstinence. Nevertheless, these
effects have been found only in heavy
drinkers. Few estimates exist for a threshold
beyond which a moderate drinker experiences
mental or neurological impairment, but a
conservative limit of 60 to 80 grams a day for
men and 30 to 50 grams a day for women
(Robertson 1984) has been suggested because
these levels are not associated with any
specific neurological deficits.

Light and moderate drinkers often are found to live longer than abstainers and heavy drinkers, according to data going back to 1926 and confirmed in long term studies involving tens of thousands of people (Breslow 1980, Gordon 1987, Klatsky 1981 and Richman 1985). Individuals in these studies who drank about one ounce of absolute ethanol a day lived longer than those who consumed greater or lesser amounts, including people who did not drink at all. In one study (Breslow 1980), limited alcohol consumption was one of a list of health habits associated with a longer life.

Healthy skepticism needed

Whatever else is taken from this text, I hope there develops in society a new skepticism about the statistics of alcohol abuse. Peter Finch, in a perceptive article called "Creative Statistics" (Health, Lifestyle and Environment 1991) makes a telling distinction between a *controller* and an *educator:*

> *The overriding aim of the health activist is action to modify human behaviour. The aim of the health educator is to tell people what they need to know in order to make informed choices for themselves.*

> *The health activist has already*
> *made those choices for us and his*
> *or her primary aim is legislation to*
> *ensure that we abide by them.*

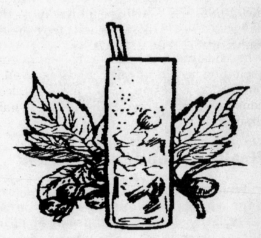

To drink or not to drink

The core problem is that the neoprohibitionists have taken over the mechanisms of public health. They are using *government* to make us do what *they* want us to do. To drink less.

Benjamin Franklin advised, "Eat not to dullness; drink not to elevation." He also wrote, "Wine is constant proof that God loves us and loves to see us happy." We recognize the serious dangers to society in abuse and how important our way of looking at these problems becomes.

In *Recent Developments in Alcoholism* (Hill 1984), the author provides the kind of encompassing, sensitive philosophy that moderates would like to see adopted by public health agencies at all levels:

> *In contrast, a third approach, which developed out of the culture of personality, places less stress on the disruptive and escapist functions of alcohol consumption and emphasizes the ways in which alcohol contributes to the maintenance of a socio-cultural system. . . . Even though some forms of heavy drinking may be perceived as deviant and disruptive, others are seen as normative and may be interpreted as modified expressions of traditional values and activities.*

These "traditional values" must be brought into consideration in government policymaking and in control practices..

Part V

The

Future

Chapter 19

One choice:
neo-prohibition

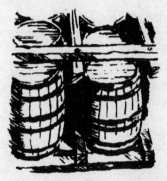

This book has explored briefly the scientific literature on drinking and health. In many chapters, it has charged that agencies of our federal government are downplaying the positive aspects of this health research because of commitments to an international movement to reduce licensed beverage consumption.

This argument is explored at length in my book *The Benefits of Moderate Drinking: Alcohol, Health and Society.* (Ford 1988) This chapter discusses the Control of Availability political agenda; shows how it is failing to reduce drinking problems; and traces its beginnings.

Here is one authority's summary of the political goals of what he calls our "third great wave of temperance" (Pittman 1988):

- *Raising the majority age to drink to twenty-one*
- *Restricting or curtailing alcohol advertising*
- *Curtailing hours of retail availability*
- *Enforcing mandatory price increases*
- *Imposing health warning labels*
- *Disallowing normal business deductions*
- *Placement of health warnings in advertising*
- *Earmarking of tax funds for treatment*
- *Tying pricing to consumer price index*
- *Raising and equalizing excise taxes*

These are all punitive goals. They are warmly supported by the National Council on Alcoholism and Drug Dependence, the Center for Science in the Public Interest and many of the hundred-odd advocacy groups brought together in neoprohibition coalitions. They are also, unfortunately, the agenda of NIAAA, OSAP and ADAMHA, the major action departments of Health and Human Services.

Political power of the drys

The anti-alcohol coalitions have had extraordinary success in about ten years of organized activity. It is frightening to acknowledge that so many of these goals have been achieved so quickly.

Congress engineered the drinking age to twenty-one by threatening states with the loss of highway grants. The Congress also succumbed to Senator Strom Thurmond's ten year campaign and decorated each liquor bottle with misleading warning messages.

Others in Congress are now proposing warnings for radio, TV and print ads despite poll evidence that over 95% of Americans are already aware of the dangers. Tax equalization is being pressed by some in a fund-hungry Congress and dozens of states have raised "sin taxes." Disallowance of advertising as a business expense is being proposed. It's a wonder that enforced pricing and shortened hours of sale have not surfaced. Control measures dominate.

Taken as a whole—as an entire agenda—there is the potential for economic devastation for the licensed beverage producing, wholesaling and retailing industries—and for many states in which they domicile. Control of Availability is Prohibition without the Eighteenth Amendment. But few in our society comprehend these perils.

It is an appalling spectacle to see a major legal industry under sustained economic attack by powerful *governmental* agencies. No business could long survive the economic constraints of the Control of Availability political agenda.

Excessive controls beget abuse

Many agencies of government today are fostering these programs despite a considerable base of research demonstrating a *negative* relationship between the severity of control laws and alcohol-related disruption (Linsky 1986, Robinson 1979 and Brenner 1987). An AMA study finds "Students get intoxicated more often and are motivated to drink to get drunk" (AMA 1992).

In a survey of the laws in all fifty states, Linsky concludes that proscriptive or punitive laws are highly correlated to *higher levels* of alcohol problems.

> *States that have the strongest*
> *cultural biases against beverage*
> *alcohol tend to be the same states*
> *that experience the most problems*
> *(i.e., the highest arrest rates*
> *associated with drinking).*

The Linsky study listed Mississippi with the most problems per capita from drinking and Nevada with the fewest. A study of nine industrialized countries traced punitive economic changes as important criteria for the incidence of abuse (Brenner 1987). Another (Dull 1986) studied alcohol-related problems in Tennessee cities of over 10,000 population where local option prevails on alcohol controls. This study concluded:

> *The findings indicate that alcohol*
> *availability measures are almost*
> *uniformly negatively correlated*
> *with the dependent variables. The*

*"forbidden fruit" concept was
advanced to explain the findings.*

Soviets gave up on controls

The most dramatic and widely publicized
failure of Control of Availability occurred in
the Soviet Union during the first five years of
the Gorbechev era. This was the perfect
laboratory. The U.S.S.R., like the U.S., was a
vast country with many ethnic and cultural
groupings. After three years of high prices
and controlled (less) availability, a sugar
shortage spread across the nation because of
moonshine production. "We must admit our
attack on drunkenness has failed," reported a
Soviet official in the December 1989 issue of
the *Economist*. The article continues:

> *A disaster it was, but one the
> Russians are learning from. They
> have become more and more aware
> of the complexity of the drink
> phenomenon, and the inadequacy
> of simple, Stalinist solutions . . . .
> Instead of waging a campaign
> against the entire population,
> efforts should be concentrated on
> the 10 percent who are alcoholics.
> The only solution is to create a
> culture of leisure.*

NIAAA and the neodry advocacy

Anti-alcoholism at the federal level did not
begin with the appointment of Dr. Ernest
Noble as second director at NIAAA. But it was
institutionalized then. As reported in the
Journal of Studies on Alcohol (Lewis 1967):

> *In a relatively brief period, Dr.
> Ernest Noble, who on February 1,
> 1976 took office as director of the
> National Institute on Alcohol
> Abuses and Alcoholism (NIAAA),
> has set a new tone and pace for the
> federal alcoholism effort.*

Noble's priority of reducing *drinking*—as
contrasted with reducing *abuse*—soon
became and still is job number-one at the
agency (Dimas 1984):

> *In June, one of the many U.S.
> government agencies involved with
> alcoholism and alcohol problems,
> the National Institute on Alcohol
> Abuse and Alcoholism, proposed
> that what is called the stabilization
> of consumption become the first
> priority of that agency.*

Ernest Noble is still at it. Though now a professor at the University of California, Noble remains active in the pursuit of his goals. In a speech to an international conference at Nice, France in 1987, Noble reiterated neoprohibition's goal of reducing consumption in the United States:

> *I feel that a realistic target will be
> to reduce per capita consumption
> by 0.1 gallon per annum so that by
> the year 2000, per capita alcohol
> consumption will be 1.4 gallons
> or the same amount as pre-World
> War II.*

Noble's legacy

Noble's legacy lives and thrives through those he brought into government. Programs were developed which carried more political thrust than scientific research or prevention programming. Here are comments:

> *What disturbs me more at the
> moment is that the distribution of
> consumption model (Control of
> Availability) is being offered as if
> it were the obvious and logical
> conclusion, even in books where the*

> *individual chapters . . . provide
> strong evidence to the contrary.
> (Heath 1988).*

Thus, the NIAAA aids the dry agenda by
channeling grants to researchers who are
supportive of the control of availability
concept and by publishing studies which
exaggerate the magnitude of alcohol-related
problems.

NIAAA radicalized

I am certain that many scientists at NIAAA
are uncomfortable with the agency's official
bias against drinking. How did an agency
designed to help the *alcoholic* and the *abuser*
become a champion of the the World Health
Organization's temperance agenda to reduce
drinking? The agency didn't begin that way.
Under the policies of its first director, Dr.
Morris Chafetz, the NIAAA had very clearly
stated policies that dignified the proper uses
of alcohol (*Second Special Report* 1974):

> *The general public should under-
> stand the facts about alcohol and
> its effects on the human body. . . .
> The proper use of alcohol can be
> socially, psychologically, and*

> *physically beneficial. . . . Those*
> *who drink should respect the*
> *decision of those who choose not to.*

Within a decade, the original policy of *responsible drinking* at NIAAA had been corrupted to the point that the longtime editor of the *Journal of Studies on Alcohol* branded the agency as inhibitionist (Keller 1985):

> *But they do recommend a policy of*
> *controls, that government should*
> *interfere with the availability of*
> *alcohol to the entire population.*
> *One critic has called this recom-*
> *mendation neoprohibition.*
> *Perhaps a more just term is*
> *"inhibition."*

From the host to the agent

This federal radicalism has been possible because there is no real advocacy in favor of drinking. Who's *for* drinking? The producing industries have been cowed by fear of lawsuits and fear of market retribution by anti-alcohol advocacies. There is no voice for reason and responsibility on drinking in Congress. Alcohol is the demon once again.

Fabricated myths and malarkey abound. As this book has shown, nearly all the statistics put out by NIAAA are questioned in the professional research—the number of alcoholics, the two-drinks-a-day heavy drinking concept, the 5,000 FAS births, and the "alcohol-involved" highway death figures. These questionable data show up in the public health literature and are repeated uncritically in the media. Control advocates, in and out of government, continue to push demonstrably false assumptions such as these non sequiturs:

> *Research has shown that increases in per capita consumption in the population will result in increased long-term health problems."*
> *(Mosher 1989).*

> *The individual (or host), alcoholic beverages (the agent) and the environment . . . (Institute on Medicine 1990).*

Control radicals—in and out of government—have successfully moved the focus from the abuser (the host drinker) to the agent (alcohol) and the environment (Mosher 1989). The NIAAA simply ignores the

accumulating research that *availability* has
little to do with *abuse*. Here are samples.

> *Neither the sales nor survey data
> supported the Distribution of
> Consumption Prevention Model
> prediction that the increased wine
> availability would produce a
> significant and lasting increase in
> wine consumption and in the
> prevalence of heavy drinkers and
> problem drinkers (Mulford 1989).*

> *It is concluded that, on the whole,
> the available evidence is too incon-
> sistent to support the control-of-
> consumption approach and that a
> more comprehensive understanding
> of alcohol abuse and prevention is
> needed (Rawn 1987).*

> *In a national sample of 3,375
> college students during the 1987-
> 1988 academic year, significantly
> more underage students were found
> to drink. This relationship is in
> marked contrast to the pattern
> documented by research extending
> back to the early 1950s and is*

*interpreted as supporting the
reactance theory (Engs 1989).*

*The social policy recommendations
of making alcoholic beverages less
available and more expensive, to
reduce per capita consumption . . .
has serious methodological
problems (Pittman 1980).*

*What is curious about recent
comments is that these benefits,
enjoyed by 90 per cent of the population, have been ridiculed or ignored
while the hazards which face only
a minority have been exaggerated
(Anderson 1989).*

No mystery in moderation

We desperately need truly temperate,
moderate lifestyle goals—to learn to pace our
drinking, to always eat when drinking, and to
set peer group standards that reinforce
sobriety as do the Jewish and Italian cultures.

Turner strongly urges the establishment
of cultural expectations that self-regulate the
parameters of social drinking. Without strong
communal constraints, drinking inevitably

becomes a menace to individuals and to the
society at large (Turner 1981):

> *Alcohol is a cultural artifact and*
> *the forms and meanings of drink-*
> *ing alcoholic beverages are cultural-*
> *ly defined. The form is usually*
> *quite explicitly stipulated, includ-*
> *ing the kind of drink that can be*
> *used, the amount and rate of*
> *intake, the time and place of*
> *drinking, the accompanying ritual,*
> *the sex and age of the drinker, and*
> *the role of behavior proper to*
> *drinking.*

You reap what you sow

Erickson in *Wayward Puritans: A Study in
the Sociology of Deviance,* characterizes
neodrys as fearful men and women—as
creators of their own demons:

> *It is not surprising that deviant*
> *behavior should seem to appear in*
> *a community at exactly those points*
> *where it is most feared. Men who*
> *fear witches soon find them-*
> *selves surrounded by them.*

Chapter 20

Another choice: the moderate middle way

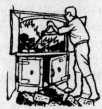

Americans are, by and large, a moderate lot. We more often take the middle way. Communism, populism, fascism—the radical super-solutions to social and political problems—have never succeeded here.

This book began with the premise that the French paradox was not quite as mysterious as our larger failure to resolve the role of drinking in society. In a perceptive assessment of our "demon drink" syndrome, London's Jancis Robinson questions America's obsession (Robinson 1988):

> *In so many aspects of social life, the
> United States of America is very
> like Britain. In terms of attitudes to
> drink, however, the Atlantic repre-
> sents a perceptible, often baffling,
> sometimes regrettable divide.
> Current American concern, one
> might say almost preoccupation,
> with personal health has yielded a
> crop of worrying medical "dis-
> coveries."*

The gospel of neodry advocacy is found in
"New Directions In Alcohol Policy" (Mosher
and Jernigan 1989). Drys today utilize
sophisticated public information techniques
and clever advocacy coalitions to achieve
punitive laws and controls. Mosher writes:

> *State and local campaigns both
> feed into and draw from efforts at
> the federal level. CSPI (Center for
> Science in the Public Interest) and
> NCA (National Council on
> Alcoholism) have led the way in
> organizing two major national
> coalitions, the National Alcohol
> Tax Commission (NATC) and
> PROJECT SMART. NATC brought
> the American Association of*

> *Retired Persons, the Association of*
> *Junior Leagues, the Children's*
> *Defense Fund, the National*
> *Women's Health Fund, and over*
> *25 other major national*
> *organizations together on behalf*
> *of excise tax increases.*

This is high visibility, media-oriented, coalition politics. The irony is that these efforts are often supported and funded by HHS, the largest health bureaucracy in the world. The sensible way to countermand this minority movement is to form state coalitions of farmers, producers, union workers, wholesalers, suppliers, tourism executives—all those forces which will be severely impacted if the dry coalitions achieve their goal of a 25% reduction in drinking.

There is an alternative. It is to enact the responsible drinking recommendations of the Education Commission of the States study *Responsible Decisions About Alcohol*.

The fundamental question is not whether drinking is *good* for heart health—though there is an abundance of medical research that says so. The real question is whether an anti-drinking minority should control the federal health bureaucracy and to discredit important health data (Tremper in Roman 1991) and to misuse it for political purposes:

> *Results of epidemiological study,
> evaluation and other research are
> adopted or adapted and selectively
> used to bolster positions and supprt
> conclusions already made. Results
> that do not fit the field's needs or
> preconceptions are ignored or,
> worse yet, atttacked and
> discredited.*

To counter this insidious bureaucratic health corruption, I suggest that Congress mandate a "middle way" agenda:

1. Eliminate completely the deceptive "alcohol and drugs" linkage.

2. Replace the anti-drinking goals in *Healthy People 2000* with the moderate goals set forth in the *ECS Responsible Decisions About Alcohol.*

3. Renew the cooperation between government, industry and private groups to reduce alcohol abuse and drunken driving.

4. Research the benefits of responsible drinking along with costs of abuse.

Text References

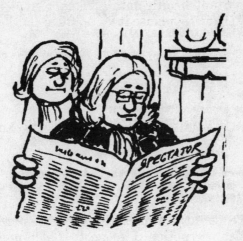

Abel, E., Fetal Alcohol Syndrome, Medical Economics Books, Oradel, 1990

Abel, E., and Sokol, R., A Revised Conserative Estimate of the Incidence of FAS and its Economic Impact, Alcohol, Clinical & Experimental Research, 15(3) June, 1991

ADAMHA NEWS, The Secretary's Program, January 1988

Akers, R, and La Greca, A, Alcohol Use Among the Elderly: Social Learning Community Context and Life Events, in Society, Culture and Drinking Patterns Reexamined, Rutgers Center for Alcohol Studies, New Brunswick 1991

Alcohol and Alcoholism, National Institute of Mental Health, Chevy Chase, Maryland, 1987

Alcohol Problems: A Report to the Nation, Oxford University Press, New York, 1987

Alcohol-Related Programs in Scandinavia Compared, ADAMHA NEWS, January/February 1989

Alcohol Report, ADAMHA NEWS, USDHHS, Vol. 13, No. 4, 1987

American Adults, Circulation 74 (6), 1465A-1468A, 1986

American Council on Science and Health, Mother Nature and Her Chemicals, News Release, New York, November 20, 1987

American Council on Science and Health, The Responsible Use of Alcohol: Defining the Parameters of Moderation, American Council on Science and Health, New York, 1991

American Heart Association, Annual Heart and Blood Vessel Disease Deaths Far Exceed The Total of Last Four Major Wars, News Release, NR 88-3672, January 18, 1988

American Heart Association, Drink a Little and Help Your Heart? Scientists Find Possible Reasons, News Release, NR 87-3657, November 19, 1987 (Hennekens/Buring)

American Heart Association, 1988 Heart Facts Reference Sheet, Dallas, 1988

American Heart Association, Two Roads to High Blood Pressure in Women: Alcohol, Lack of 2 Minerals, New Release, NR 87-3642, November 16, 1987 (Witteman/Hennekens)

American Medical Association, Manual on Alcoholism, 1986

American Medical Association, Traffic Deaths Down But Costs Still Staggering, News Release July 14, 1992

American Public Health Association, Alcohol Tax Policy Reform, Washington, D.C., 1987

Ames, B., Cancer Scares Over Trivia, Los Angeles Times, Thursday, May 15, 1986

Ames, B., Magaw, R., and Gold, L., Ranking Possible Carcinogenic Hazards, Science, Vol., 236, 1987

Anderson, D., Ed., Drinking to Your Health, Social Affairs Unit, London 1989

Asch, P., and Levy, D., The Minimum Legal Drinking Age and Traffic Fatalities, National Institute on Alcohol Abuse and Alcoholism, Washington, D.C., November, 1986

Babor, T., Kranzler, H., and Lauerman, R., Social Drinking as a Health and Psychosocial Risk Factor: Anstie's Limit Revisited, Recent Developments in Alcoholism, Edited by Marc Galanter, Plenum Press, New York, 1987

Barsby, S., Societal costs of alcohol abuse still overstated, The Moderation Reader, March/April, 1991

BATF, Letter from T. Skora to Leeward Winery, 1992

Bertels, T., In Pursuit of Agri-Power, Silver Lake College Press, 1988

Boffetta, P., and Garfinkel, L., Alcohol Drinking and Mortality Among Men Enrolled in an American Cancer Society Prospective Study, Epidemiology, V.1, No. 5, 1990

Bottom Line, Alcohol Problems Around the World, Spring, 1987

Bottom Line, New Developments in the Battle for Stomach Share, and U.S. Charitable Giving Hits Record High, Winter, 1987

Bottom Line, Statistical Review, Fall, 1987

Bowden, S., Cerebral Deficits in Social Drinkers and the Onus of Proof, Australian Drug and Alcohol Review, 1987:6: 98-92

Bowen, O., Remarks to the National Conference on Alcohol Abuse and Alcoholism, DHHS, Washington, D.C., November 12, 1987

Brenner, M., Economic Change, Alcohol Consumption and Heart Disease Mortalilty in Nine Industrialized Countries, Social Science Medicine, Vol. 25, No. 2, 119-132, 1987

Breslow, L., and Enstrom, J., Persistence of Health Habits and Their Relationship to Mortality, Preventive Medicine 9: 469-483m 1980

Cahalan, D., Understanding America's Drinking Problem, Jossey-Bass Publishers, San Francisco, 1987

Camargo, C. A., et al. The Effect of Moderate Alcohol Intake on Serum Apolipoproteins, A-I and A-II. Journal of the American Medical Association 253(19): 2854-2857, 1985

Castelli, W., Epidemiology of Coronary Heart Disease: The Framingham Study, The American Journal of Medicine, February 27, 1984

Centers for Disease Control, Telephone Survey, February 12, 1987

Chafetz, M., Why Drinking Can Be Good For You, Stein and Day, New York, 1976

Chalke, H.D., Moderate Drinking-Moderate Damage, British Journal on Alcohol and Alcoholism, Vol. 16, No. 3, 1981

Choi, S, et al., Effect of cigarette smoking and alcohol consumption in the etiology of cancers of the digestive tract, Internal Journal of Cancer 49(3), September 1991

Cohn, V., Reporting on Risk, The Media Institute, Washington, D.C., 1990

Colquitt, M., Fielding L., and Cronan J., Drunk Drivers and Medical and Social Injury, New England Journal of Medicine, Vol. 317, No. 20, November, 1987

Cope, G, et al., Alcohol consumption in patients with colorectal adenomatous polyps, Gut, January 1991

Cowan, R., and Mosher, J., Public Health Implications of Beverage Marketing, Contemporary Drug Problems, Winter 1985

Davis, R., Alcohol and Agriculture: Their Shared Threats, Speech, 1988

DeLabry, L., et al., Alcohol consumption and mortality in an American male population, Journal of Studies on Alcohol, 53(1), 1992

Demographic Trends, Alcohol Abuse and Alcoholism, NIAAA Epidemiological Bulletin No. 15, Vol. 5, Spring 1987

Department of Health and Human Services, My Baby. . . Strong and Healthy, U.S. Government Printing Office, Washington,D.C.

Department of Health and Human Services, Second Special Report to Congress on Alcohol and Health, June, 1974

Department of Health and Human Services, Surveillance Report No. 7, Apparent Per Capita Alcohol Consumption, National, State and Regional Trends, Washington, D.C., September, 1987

Dimas, G., Rebuilding an American Consensus for Alcoholism, The U.S. Journal, November 1984

Dolnick, E., Le Paradoxe Francaise, In Health, May/June, 1990

Donohue, R. P., et al., Alcohol and Hemorrhagic Stroke: The Honolulu Heart Program, Journal of the American Medical Association 255 (17): 2311-2314, 1986

Dorris, M., The Broken Cord, Harper and Row, New York, 1989

Douglas, M., Ed., Constructive Drinking, Cambridge University Press, New York, 1987

Drinking and Crime, National Institute of Justice, USDJ, Washington, D.C. 1990

Drunk Driving Facts, NHTSA, Washington, D.C., 1988

Dull, R., and Giocopasso, D., An Assessment of the Effects of Alcohol Ordinances on Selected Behaviors and Conditions, The Journal of Drug Issues, 16(4), pp 511-521, 1986

Easterbrook, G., Everything You Know About the Environment is Wrong, New Republic, April 30, 1990

Eckhard, M., et al., Health Hazards Associated with Alcohol Consumption, Journal of the American Medical Association, Vol. 246, No. 6, 1981

Education Commission of the States Program on Drinking and Pregnancy, Washington, D.C., 1980

Education Commission of the States, Interim Report Number 4, Denver 1975

Ellison, C., Benefits of a little wine should not be lost in efforts to curb abuse, Medical World News, December 1990

Ellison, C., Speech to AWARE Seminar, Philadelphia, May 4, 1990

Emboden, W., "Natural Highs" in an Historical and Biological Context, Journal of Drug Education, Vol 18, (1), 1988

Farrell, S., Review of National Policy Measures to Prevent Alcohol-Related Problems, World Health Organization, Geneva, 1985

Engs, R., and Hanson, D., Reactance Theory: A Test with Collegiate Drinking, Psychological Reports, Vol. 64, 1989

Erickson, K., Wayward Puritans: A Study in the Sociology of Deviance, John Wiley & Sons, New York, 1966

Ewing, J., and Rouse, B., Drinking, Nelson Hill, Chicago, 1978

Ferrence, R., Truscott, S., and Whitehead, P., Drinking and the Prevention of Coronary Heart Disease: Findings, Issues and Public Health Policy, Journal of Studies on Alcohol, Vol. 47, No. 5, 1986

Fingarette, H., Heavy Drinking, University of California Press, Berkeley, 1988

Forsham, P., The Impact of Wine on Diabetes Mellitus, Bulletin of the Medical Friends of Wine, Vol. 29, No. 1, 1987

Fraenkel-Conrat, H., and Singer, B., Nucleoside adducts are formed by cooperative reaction of acetaldehyde and alcohols: Possible mechanism for the role of ethanol in carcinogenesis, Proceedings of the National Academy of Sciences, Vol. 85, 3758-3761, June 1988

Franke G., and Wilcox, G., Alcoholic Beverage Advertising and Consumption in the United States, 1964-1984, Journal of Advertising, Vol. 16, No. 3, 1987, 22-30

Fraser, G, Eating Nuts May Reduce the Risk of Coronary Heart Disease, AMA News Release, Chicago July 15, 1992

Fredda, M., et al., High Blood Alcohol Levels in Women, New England Journal of Medicine, Vol. 322, No. 2, January, 1990

Friedman, L., and Kimball, A., Coronary Heart Disease, Mortality and Alcohol Consumption in Framingham, American Journal of Epidemiology, 1983.

Gastineau, C., Darby, and Turner, T., Fermented Food Beverages in Nutrition, New York, Academic Press, Inc., 1979

Gavalier,L, and Van Thiel, D, The Association Between Moderate Alcohol Beverage Consumption and Serum Estradiol and Testasterone Levels in Normal Menopausal Women: Relationship to the Literature of Alcohol, Clinical and Experimental Research, V.6(1) 1992

Gentry, K., The Christian and Alcoholic Beverages, Baker Book House, Grand Rapids, 1986

Ghadirian, P., et al., Tobacco, alcohol, and coffee and cancer of the pancreas, A population -based, case control study in Quebec, Cancer 67(10) May 1991

Gill, J., et al., Alcohol consumption—a risk factor for hemorrhagic and non-hemorrhagic stroke, American Journal of Medicine, 90(4), April 1990

Gill, J., et. al. Stroke and Alcohol Consumption, New England Journal of Medicine 315 (17): 1041-1046, 1986.

Gilson, C., Progress & Potential, The ACA Journal, Summer/Fall, 1989

Gilson, C., Women v. men . . . and moderate levels of drinking, Moderation Reader, Seattle, July/August, 1991

Gleiberman, L., and Harburg, E. Alcohol Usage and Blood Pressure: A Review. Human Biology 58(1): 1-31, 1986

Goldstein, D., Pharmacology of Alcohol, Oxford University Press, New York, 1983

Gordis, E., Alcoholism: A Family Legacy?, ADAMHA NEWS, Vol. XIII, No. 6, June, 1987

Gordis, E., Confronting Alcohol Abuse and Dependence, ADAMHA NEWS, January-February 1980

Gordis, E, Moderate Drinking, Alcohol Alert, NIAAA, April 1991

Gordon, T., and Doyle, J. Drinking and Mortality: The Albany Study, American Journal of Epidemiology 125(2): 263-270, 1987

Gordon, T., and Kannell, W., Drinking Habits and Cardiovascular Disease: The Framingham Study, American Heart Journal, 105 (4): , 1983

Graham, J., et al., Independent Dysmorphology Evaluation at Birth and 4 Years of Age for Children Exposed to Varying Amounts of Alcohol in Utero, Pediatrics,Vol. 81, No. 6, June, 1988

Graham, S., Alcohol and Breast Cancer, New England Journal of Medicine 316 (9): 1211-1212, 1987

Grant, M., Preventing Alcohol Abuse, Testimony to the U.S. Senate, WHO, 1988

Gray, W., "Koop crusade" rolls on with disturbing leadership mix, Moderation Reader, November/December, 1990

Grossarth-Maticek, R., et al., Personality, stress and motivational factors in drinking as determinants of risk for cancer and coronary heart disease, Psychological Reports, 69(3), December 1991

Gruchow, H., et al. Effects of Drinking Patterns on the Relationship Between Alcohol and Coronary Occlusion. Atherosclerosis 43: 393-4041988

Gunby, P., Alcoholism Research Report Acknowledges Progress, Emphasizes Need to Understand Underlying Pathology, Assess Treatment Results, Journal of American Medical Association 257(21): 2876-2877, 1987

Gusfield, J., The Culture of Public Problems, University of Chicago Press, 1981

Gusfield, J., et. al., The Social Control of Drinking-Driving: An Ethnographic Study of Bar Settings, Law & Policy, Vol. 6, January, 1984

Hamelsmaki, et al., Patterns of Consumption During Pregnancy, Obstetrics and Gynecology, 1987

Harburg, E., Davis, D., and Caplan, R., Parent and Offspring Alcohol Use, Journal of Studies on Alcohol, Vol. 43, No. 5, 1982

Harris, L., Inside America, Vintage Books, New York, 1988

Harris, R., and Wynder, E., Breast Cancer and Alcohol Consumption, Journal of the American Medical Association, Vol. 259, No. 9, May 20, 1989

Harvey, E. B., Schairer, C., Brinton, L. A., et. al. Alcohol Consumption and Breast Cancer. Journal of the National Cancer Institute 78(4): 667-661, 1987

Haskell, W., et al. The Effect of Cessation and Resumption of Moderate Alcohol Intake on Serum High-density-Lipoprotein Subfractions, New England Journal of Medicine 310 (13): 805-810, 1984

Health and Human Services, Seventh Special Report to Congress on Alcohol and Health, Washington, D.C.

Healthy Public Policy, Briefing Paper, Australian Wine and Brandy Producers, Adelaide, 1988

Heath, D., A Decade of Development in the Anthropological Study of Alcohol Use, in Constructive Drinking, Douglas, M., editor, Cambridge University Press, N.Y., 1987

Heath, D., Alcohol Control Policies and Drinking Patterns: An International Game of Politics Against Science, Journal of Substance Abuse, 1, 109-111, 1988

Heath, D., Alcohol Use, 1970-1980, in Constructive Drinking, editor, Douglas, M., Cambridge University Press, Cambridge, 1987

Heath, D., Quasi-Science and Public Policy: A Reply to Robin Room about Details and Misrepresentations in Science, Journal of Substance Abuse, 1, 121-125, 1988

Heath, D., and Cooper, A., Lesson on Drinking: The Italians Can Do It Best, The Wall Street Journal, January 13, 1988

Heien D, Pompelli, G, Stress, Ethnic and Distribution Factors in a Dichotomous Response Model of Alcohol Abuse, Journal of Studies on Alcohol, Vol. 48, 1987

Hennekens, C., American Heart Association, News Release, Abstract #1990, Dallas, November 19, 1987

Herbert, V., et al., Alcohol and Breast Cancer. New England Journal of Medicine 317: 1287-1288, 1987

Hewlett, A., An alternative to neo-prohibition, Moderation Reader, November/December, 1991

Hewlett, A., How federal neo-prohibition was launched by Dr. Ernest Noble, Moderation Reader, May/June, 1990

Hiatt, R., et al., Alcohol Consumption and the Risk of Breast Cancer in a Prepaid Health Plan, Cancer Research 48, (8): 2284-2287, 1988

Hill, T., in Recent Developments in Alcoholism, Galanter, M., Ed., Plenum Press, New York, 1984

Hilton M., and Clark, W., Changes in American Drinking Patterns and Problems, 1967-1984, Journal of Studies on Alcohol, Vol. 48, No.6, 1987

Hilton, M., and Kosbutas, L., Public support for warning labels on alcoholic beverage containers, British Journal of Addiction, 86(10), October 1991

Holder, H., Prevention of Alcohol-Related Problems, Alcohol, Health and Research World, Vol. 13, No. 4, 339-342, 1989

Holmgren, E., Health Issues, Wines and Vines, June 1992

Huber, P., Liability: The Legal Revolution and its Consequences, Basic Books, New York, 1988

Inner City Youth: A Challenge for Drug Prevention Efforts, ADAMHA NEWS, Vol. 14, No. 4, April, 1988

Jackson, R., et al., Alcohol consumption and risk of coronary heart disease, British Medical Journal, 303, July 27, 1991

Jellinek E. M., The Symbolism of Drinking; A Cultural-Historical Approach, Journal of Studies on Alcohol, Vol. 38, 852-856, 197

Johnson, E., Letter to Gene Ford, Moderation Reader, January/February, 1992

Johnston, L.,Illicit Drug Use by American High School Seniors Resumed its Gradual Decline in 1986, but Not Among Cocaine Users, Institute for Social Research, University of Michigan, February 20, 1987

Josephson, E., and Haberman, P., Assessment of Statistics on Alcohol-Related Problems, Columbia University School of Public Health, New York, 1980

Kaplan, N., Bashing booze: the danger of losing the benefits of moderate alcohol consumption, American Heart Journal, June 1991

Karen, G., and Klein N., Bias against negative studies in newspaper reports of medical research, Journal of American Medical Association, 2267, 1991

Kastenbaum, R., Generations, Summer 1988

Katz, P., Bulletin, The Beer Institute, Washington, D.C., 1987

Katz, S., Speech to AWARE Seminar, Philadelphia, May 5, 1990

Katz, S., and Voight, M. M., Bread and Beer, Expeditions, 29(2):2, 1986

Keller, M., Alcohol Problems and Policies, in Law, Alcohol, and Order, Edited by Kyvig, D., Greenwood Press, Westport, 1985

Kelsey, J., and Berkowitz, G., Breast Cancer Epidemiology, Cancer Research, 48:5615-5623, 1988

Kendell, R. E., et. al., Drinking Sensibly, British Journal of Addiction, 82 & 83, 1987

Klatsky, A., Alcohol and Cardiovascular Disorders: Abstinence May Be Hazardous to Some Persons, Speech to National Press Club, June 10, 1991

Klatsky, A., Armstrong, M., and Friedman, G., Relations of Alcoholic Beverage Use to Subsequent Coronary Artery Disease Hospitalization, Journal of Cardiology 58: 710-714, 1986

Klatsky, A., Friedman, G., and Siegelaub, A., Alcohol and Mortality: A Ten-Year Kaiser-Permanente Experience. Annals of Internal Medicine 95 (2): 139-145, 1981

Klatsky, A., Friedman, G., and Siegelaub, A., Alcohol Use and Cardiovasclar Disease: The Kaiser-Permanente Experience, Circulation 64, Supplement III, III-32-III-41, 1981.

Klein, T., DWI - Are We Off Track?, Straight Talk About Drunk Driving, Beverage Retailers Against Driving Drunk, June, 1986

Knupfer, G., Drinking for Health: The daily light drinker fiction, British Journal of Addiction, 82, 547-555, 1987

Kristol, I., The Good Life and the New Class, in Health, Lifestyle and Environment, Social Affairs Unit/Manhattan Institute, 1991

La Porte, R., Cresanta, J., and Kuller, L., The Relationship of Alcohol Consumption to Atherosclerotic Heart Disease, Preventive Medicine, 9., 22-40 (1980)

Lazarus, N., et al., Change in alcohol consumpion and risk of death from all causes and from ischaemic heart disease, British Medical Journal September 1991

Leger, A., et al., Factors Associated with Cardiac Mortalilty in Developed Countries with Particular Reference to Wine, The Lancet, May 12, 1979

Leighton, T, Presentation to the American Chemical Society Annual Meeting, 1991

Levine, H., The Alcohol Problem in America: From Temperance to Alcoholism, British Journal of Addiction, 79, 1984

Levine, H., The Committee of Fifty and the Origins of Alcohol Control, Journal of Drug Issues, 13(1), 1983

Lewis, J., Washington Report, Journal of Studies on Alcohol, Vol. 37, No. 9, 1976

Lex, B., et al., Blood Ethanol Levels, Self-Rated Ethanol Effects and Cognitive-Perceptual Tasks, Pharmacology Biochemistry & Behavior, Vol. 29, 1988

Licensed Beverage Information Council, Alcohol and Health: Education, Warning Labels and Responsibility to the Public, Washington, D.C., January, 1987

Lieber, C., To Drink (Moderately) or Not To Drink?, New England Journal of Medicine, 310(13): 846-848, March 29, 1984.

Lieber, C., Perspectives: do alcohol calories count? American Journal of Clinical Nutrition, December 1991

Linsky, A., Colby, J., Straus, M., Drinking Norms and Alcohol-Related Problems in the United States, Journal of Studies on Alcohol, No. 5, 1986

Livingston C., Straight Talk About The Drunk Driving Problem, BRADD, Washington, D.C., September, 1985

Longnecker, M., Associations between Alcoholic Beverage Consumption and Hospitalization, 1983 National Health Interview Survey, American Journal of Public Health, Vol. 78, No. 2, 1988

Luks, A., and Barbato, J., You Are What You Drink, The Stonesong Press, Villard Books, New York, 1989

Marmot, M., et al., Alcohol and cardiovascular disease and the status of the U-shaped curve, British Medical Journal September 7, 1991

Marshall, M., editor, Beliefs, Behaviors, & Alcoholic Beverages, the University of Michigan Press, Ann Arbor, 1979

McConnell, C., and McConnell, M., The Mediterranean Diet, W. W. Norton & Co., New York, 1987

Mendelson, J., and Mello, N., Alcohol: Use and Abuse in America, Boston: Little, Brown, and Company, 1985

Mills, J., and Grauberd, B., Is Moderate Drinking During Pregnancy Associated with an Increased Risk for Malformations, Pediatrics 80, 1987

Mishara, B., and Kastenbaum, R., Alcohol and Old Age, Grune & Stratton, New York, 1888

Moore, D., Liver Disorders, ADAMHA NEWS, USDHHS, Vol. 13, No. 6, June, 1987

Moore, D., Many Gastric Disorders Traced to Overuse of Alcohol, ADAMHA NEWS, USDHS, Vol. 13, No. 5, May, 1987

Moore, R., and Pearson, T., Moderate Alcohol Consumption and Coronary Artery Disease: A Review, Medicine 65 (4): 242-267, 1986

Moore, R., Smith, C., Kuterovich, P., and Pearson, T., American Journal of Medicine: 884-890, 1988

Morse, R, Alcoholism: How Do You Get It, in Fermented Food Beverages, Academic Press, NY 1979

Mosher, J., and Colman, V., A Handbook for Action, 1989

Mosher, J., and Jernigan, D., New Directions in Alcohol Policy, Annual Review of Public Health, 10:245-79, 1989

Mothers Against Drunk Driving, ABC's of Drinking and Driving, MADD, Hurst, TX, 1971

Mulford, H., and Fitzgerald, M., Consequences of Increasing Off-premise Wine Outlets in Iowa, 1988

Mulford, H.S., and Fitzgerald, J.L., Per Capita Sales, Heavy Drinking Prevalence and Alcohol Problems in Iowa for 1958-1985, British Journal of Addictions, (1988) 83, 265-268

National Center for Statistics & Analysis, 1987 Fatality Facts, USDOT, NHTSA, October 1988

National Highway Traffic Safety Administration, Statistics, 1991

Newcomb, and Bentlow, P., Consequences of Adolescent Drug Use, Sage Publications 1989

New England Journal of Medicine, Correspondence, Alcohol and Breast Cancer, 317, (20) 1285-1289, 1987

New York Metropolitan Life, Alcohol Use in the United States, Statistical Bulletin, January/March, 1987

Nielsen, F., Effects of Dietary Boron on Mineral, Estrogen, and Testosterone Metabolism in Postmenopausal Women, FASEB, 0892-6638, 1987

Noble,E., Prevention By and For All to Make a Safer Future, The Bottom Line, 1986

Norton, R., Bartez, R., Dwyer, T., and MacMahoney S., Alcohol Consumption and the Risk of Alcohol-Related Cirrhosis in Women, British Medical Journal 295: 80-82, 1987

O'Connell, T., Mothers Can Drink in Moderation—Researchers, U.S. Journal of Drug and Alcohol Dependence, Vol. 10, No. 2, February, 1988

Office of Substance Abuse Prevention, Communicating About Alcohol and Other Drugs: Strategies for Reaching Populations at Risk, Rockville,

Oldenburg, R., The Great Good Place, Paragon House, New York, 1989

Olsen, R., Wine and Health, Society of Wine Educators Bulletin, 1985

O'Neill, B., Speech to College of American Pathologists, Washington, D.C., 1987

OSAP, Prevention Monograph 5, Communications About Alcohol and Other Drugs, USDHHS, Rockville,

Ottoboni, M., The Dose Makes the Poison, Vincent Books, Berkeley, 1984

Peele, S., The Limitations of Control-of-Supply Models for Explaining and Preventing Alcoholism and Drug Addiction, Journal of Studies on Alcohol, Vol. 48, No. 1, 1987

Peele, S., What Does Addiction Have To Do With The Level of Consumption: A Response to Robin Room, Journal of Studies on Alcohol, Vol 48, No. 1, 1987

Per Capita Alcoholic and Nonalcoholic Beverage Consumption, Monday Morning Report, Vol. 13, No. 14, April, 1990

Pisano, S., and Rooney, J., Children's Changing Attitudes Regarding Alcohol: A Cross-Sectional Study, Journal on Drug Education, 18(1), 1988

Pisani, V., The DUI Offender, in Zeroing In On Repeat Offenders, Proceedings of the National Commission Against Drunk Driving Conference on Recidivism, September 16, 1986

Pittman, D. J., Drinking Sensibly, British Journal of Addiction, 82, 1289-1300, 1987

Pittman, D., Primary Prevention of Alcohol Abuse and Alcoholism, Social Science Institute, Washington University, St. Louis, 1980

Pittman, D., The Benefits of Moderate Drinking, Wine Appreciation Guild, San Francisco, 1988

Pittman D., and White, H., Society, Culture and Drinking Patterns Reexamined, Rutgers Center for Alcohol Studies, New Brunswick, 1991

Plant, M., Women, Drinking and Pregnancy, 1987

Plaut, T., Alcohol Problems: A Report to the Nation, Oxford University Press, New York, 1967

Pollack, E. S., et. al. Prospective Study of Alcohol Consumption and Cancer, New England Journal of Medicine 310, 617-621, 1984

Prevention and Treatment of Alcohol Problems, Research Opportunities, Institute of Medicine, Washington, D.C., 1990

Public Policy on Alcohol Problems, Sixty-Sixth American Assembly, Columbia University, Arden House, New York, April 26-29, 1984

Ramon, M., ed., Alcohol: The Development of Sociological Perspectives on Use and Abuse, Rutgers Center for Alcohol Studies, New Brunswick, 1991

Rawn, I., The Control-of-Consumption Approach to Alcohol Abuse Prevention. II. A Review of Empirical Studies, The International Journal of the Addictions, 22(10), 957-979, 1987

Renaud, S, and DeLageril, M, Wine, Alcohol, Platelets and the French Paradox for Coronary Heart Disease, The Lancet, V. 339, June 1992

Richman, A., and Warren, R. A. Alcohol Consumption and Morbidity in the Canada Health Survey: Inter-Beverage Differences, Drug and Alcohol Dependence 15: 255-282, 1985.

Rimm, E., et al., Prospective Study of Alcohol Consumption and Risk of Coronary Heart Disease in Men, Lancet 338, August 1991

Robertson, I., Does Moderate Drinking Cause Mental Impairment? British Medical Journal 289 (6447): 711-712, 1984.

Robinson, D., Drinking Behavior in Alcoholism In Perspective, Grant, M., and Gwinner, P., Croom Helm, London, 1979

Robinson, J., On the Demon Drink, Mitchell Beasley, London, 1988

Rohan, T., and McMichael, A., Alcohol Consumption and the Risk of Breast Cancer, International Journal of Cancer:41, 695-699, 1988

Room, R., Alcohol Control, Addiction and Processes of Change, Journal of Studies on Aicohol, Vol. 48 (1) 1987

Room, R., Science is in the Details: Towards a Nuanced View of Alcohol Control Studies, Journal of Substance Abuse, 1, 117-120, 1988

Rorabaugh, W., The Alcoholic Republic, Oxford University Press, New York, 1979

Rosett, H., and Weiner, L., Alcohol and the Fetus: A Clinical Perspective, Oxford University Press, 1984

Rosett, H., et al., Patterns of Alcohol Consumption and Fetal Development, Journal of the American College of Obstetricians and Gynecologists, Vol. 61, No. 5, 1983

Ross, H., Deterring the Drinking Driver, Lexington Books, Lexington, 1984

Ross, H., and Hughes, G., Drunk Driving: What Not to Do, The Nation, December 13, 1986

Rubin, E., An Overview of the Evidence Concerning the Hypothesis that Alcohol Causes Cancer, Presentation to the Scientific Committee for Proposition 65, California, published by The Wine Institute, San Francisco, 1988

St. Leger, A., Cochrane, A., and Moore, F., Factors Associated with Cardiac Mortality in Developed Countries with Particular Reference to the Consumption of Wine, The Lancet, May 12, 1979

Sankaran, H, et al., Carbohydrates Intake Determines Pancreatic Acinar Amylase Activity and Release Despite Chronic Alcoholemic In Rats, In press, American Institute of Nutrition, Accepted April 29, 1992

Sarley, V., and Stepto, R., Wine is Fine for Patients 'Morale and Helps Stimulate their Appetites, Modern Nursing Home, January/February, Vol. 23, No. 1, 1969

Schade, C., The Drug War: The Wrong Effort Aimed at Lesser Problems, The Nation's Health, March 1990

Schaefer, J., On The Potential Health Effects of Consuming "Non-Alcoholic" or "De-Alcoholized" Beverages, Alcohol, Vol. 4, 1986

Schatzkin, A., et al., Alcohol consumption and breast cancer: A cross-national correlation study, International Journal of Epidemiology, 18:28-31, 1989

Schatzkin, A., et. al,. Alcohol Consumption and Breast Cancer in the Epidemiologic Follow-Up Study of the First National Health and Nutrition Examination Survey. New England Journal of Medicine 316 (9): 1169-1173, 1987

Schenker, S., and Speeg, K., Risk of Alcohol Intake in Men and Women, New England Journal of Medicine, Vol. 322, No. 2, January, 1990

Scoles, P., Fine, E., and Steer, R., Personality Characteristics and Drinking Patterns of High-Risk Drivers Never Apprehended for Driving While Intoxicated, Journal of Studies on Alcohol, Vol. 45, No. 5, 1984

Second Special Report to the U. S. Congress on Alcohol and Health, USDHHS, 1974

Selzer R, Mortal Lessons: Notes on the Art of Surgery, Simon & Schuster, New York, 1976

Seventh Special Report to the U.S. Congress on Alcohol and Health, USDHHS, 1990

Sherman, L., Drunk Driving Tests in Fatal Accidents, Crime Control Reports, Washington, D. C., December, 1986

Shoemaker, W., Failure to diagnose properly: the under-reporting factor in FAS, Moderation Reader, May/June, 1991

Siemann, E., and Creasy, L., Concentration of the Phytoalexin Resveratrol in Wine, American Journal on Enology and Viticulture, 43(1) 1992

Simon, M., et al., Alcohol consumption and the risks of breast cancer, Journal of Clinical Epidemiology, 44(8) 1991

Simpson, H, and Mayhew, D, The Hard Core Drinking Driver, Traffic Injury Research Foundation of Canada, Ottawa 1991

Sixth Special Report to the U. S. Congress on Alcohol and Health, USDHHS, 1987

Smith, R., et al., Legislation Raising the Legal Drinking Age in Massachusetts from 18 to 20: Effect on 16 and 17 Year Olds, Journal of Studies on Alcohol, Vol. 45, No. 6, 1984

Sokol, R., as quoted in Beverage Retailers Against Drunk Driving Bulletin, July 20, 1987

Stall, R., Research Issues Concerning Alcohol Consumption Among Aging Populations, Journal. of Studies on Alcohol, Vol. 19, No. 3, May, 1987

Stamler, J., Coronary Heart Disease: Doing the "Right Things," The New England Journal of Medicine, Vol. 312, No. 16, 1986

Status Report, Myths and Misconceptions About 55 MPH Speed Limit, April 26, 1986

Steinbrook, R., Research Links Enzymes to Alcohol's Effect on Women, Los Angeles Times, January 11, 1990

Task Force on Responsible Decisions on Alcohol, Final Report, Education Conference of the States, Washington, D.C., 1977

Taylor, R., Health Fact, Health Fiction, Taylor Publishing Co., Dallas 1990

Tierney, J., Not To Worry, Hippocrates, January/February, 1988

Tomenaga, K., et al., A case-control study of stomach cancer and its genesis in relation to alcohol consumption, smoking and familial cancer history, Japanese Journal of Cancer Research 82(9) September 1991

Trebach, A., The Great Drug War, McMillan Publishing Company, New York, 1987

Turner, T, Alcohol-Related Problems in Perspective, MBAA Technical Quarterly 21(4): 171-174, 1984.

Turner, T., Mezey, E., and Kimball, A.W. Measurement of Alcohol-Related Effects in Man, Chronic Effects in Relation to Levels of Alcohol Consumption, Parts A and B.,The Johns Hopkins Medical Journal 141, 235-248 and 273-286, 1977

Turner, T. B., Bennett, V. L. and Hernandez, H., The Beneficial Side Effects of Moderate Alcohol Use. The Johns Hopkins Medical Journal 148 (2): 53, 1981

Vaillant, T, The Natural History of Alcoholism, Harvard University Press, 1983

Vogler, R., and Bartz, W., The Better Way to Drink, Simon & Schuster, New York, 1982

Vogler, R, and Bartz, W, Teenagers & Alcohol, The Charles Press, Philadelphia 1992

Wagenaar, A., Alcohol, Young Drivers, and Traffic Accidents, Lexington Books, Lexington, 1983

Walpole, I., et al., How to moderate maternal use before and during pregnancy and neurobehavioral outcome in the newborn infant, Developmental Medicine and Child Neurology 33(10) 1991

Webb, S., Hochberg, M., and Sher, M., Fetal Alcohol Syndrome: Report of Case, Journal of American Dental Association, Vol. 116, February 1988

Webster, L., et. al. Alcohol Consumption and Risk of Breast Cancer, The Lancet (1): 724-726, 1983

Weiner, C., The Politics of Alcoholism, Transaction Books, New Brunswick, 1985

Whelan, E., Consumerism and the Misdirected War Against Alcohol Advertising, Speech, DISCUS, Boca Raton, 1984

Whelan, E., Moderate drinking: how much is too much, Moderation Reader, July/August, 1991

Whelan, E., To Your Health, Across the Board, New York, January, 1983

Whitten, D., Wines Institute Seminar, San Francisco, 1987

Wiley, J., and Camachc, T., Life-Style and Future Health: Evidence from the Alameda County Study, Preventive Medicine, 9, 1-21, 1980

Willett, W. C., et. al. Moderate Alcohol Consumption and the Risk of Breast Cancer, New England Journal of Medicine, 316(9), 1174-1180, 1987

Williams A., et al., Drugs in Fatally Injured Young Male Drivers, Public Health Reports, Insurance Institute for Highway Safety, Washington, D.C., October, 1984

Williamson, D., Survey shows heavy drinking varies widely from state to state, The Seattle Times, February 13, 1987

Wine and Medical Practice, Tenth Edition, The Wine Institute, San Francisco, 1979

Wittman, F., Shane, P., Manual for Community Planning to Prevent Problems of Alcohol Availability, California State Department of Alcohol and Drug Programs, September 1988

World Health Organization, The Adelaide Recommendations, World Health Policy, April 9, 1988

Zinberg, N., Drug, Set and Setting, Yale University Press, New Haven, 1984

Zucker, R., and Noll, R., Precursors and Developmental Influences on Drinking and Alcoholism: Etiology from a Longitudinal Perspective, Alcohol Consumption and Related Problems, USDHHS, Washington, D.C., 1982

Zylman, R., A Critical Evaluation of the Literature on Alcohol Involvement in Highway Deaths, Accident, Analysis and Prevention, Vol. 6, 163-204, 1974

It's been written . . .

. . . attention came to be focused on the thing, alcohol, rather than on the people who used or abused it. So alcohol the thing was seen as the enemy. . . . And it was metamorphosed as the Demon Rum.

Mark Keller, "Alcohol Problems and Policies in Historical Perspective," in **Law Alcohol and Order,** *Greenwood Press, Westport, 1985*

Index

A

D

E

K

L

M

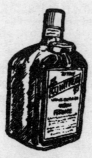

America has a serious alcohol problem, says Gene Ford, endangering the nation's health, economy, and political morality. And that problem is the "healthocrats" who want to make Americans stop drinking.

Tessa De Carlo,
American Wine & Food

The author details the many half-truths and innuendos that get ink and airtime and identifies this consortia of alcohol baiters as the Prohibition Coalition.

Patricia Kennedy,
The Alcoholic Beverage Newsletter

He stands alone on his soapbox, wishing someone would join him. It's not that nobody agrees with him, says Gene Ford. It's just that nobody wants to say so. Imbibing alcoholic beverages is fine and even healthy, insists Ford. Drinking rarely harms anyone who isn't alcoholic.

Loriannne Denne,
The Business Journal

There is probably nobody on the industry scene today who knows more about the unwarranted social pressures being put on the beverage alcohol business than Gene Ford, and nobody more willing to talk about them.

Perry Luntz,
Southern Beverage Journal

Rev. Walker had brought along prepared benediction remarks but something in Gene Ford's commencement address caused him to redraft it. Gene, an immensely popular professor, was telling them something from his heart—about how he felt that the preparation and serving of food and drink was a part of the life-giving process.

—James McCusker
Everett Herald

Both the public at large and the health-care profession must continue to do everything possible to prevent alcohol abuse. At the same time, it is essential not to prohibit or impede the continued healthful consumption of moderate amounts of alcohol.

—Norman M. Kaplan, M.D
American Heart Association, Past President